Restorative
yoga

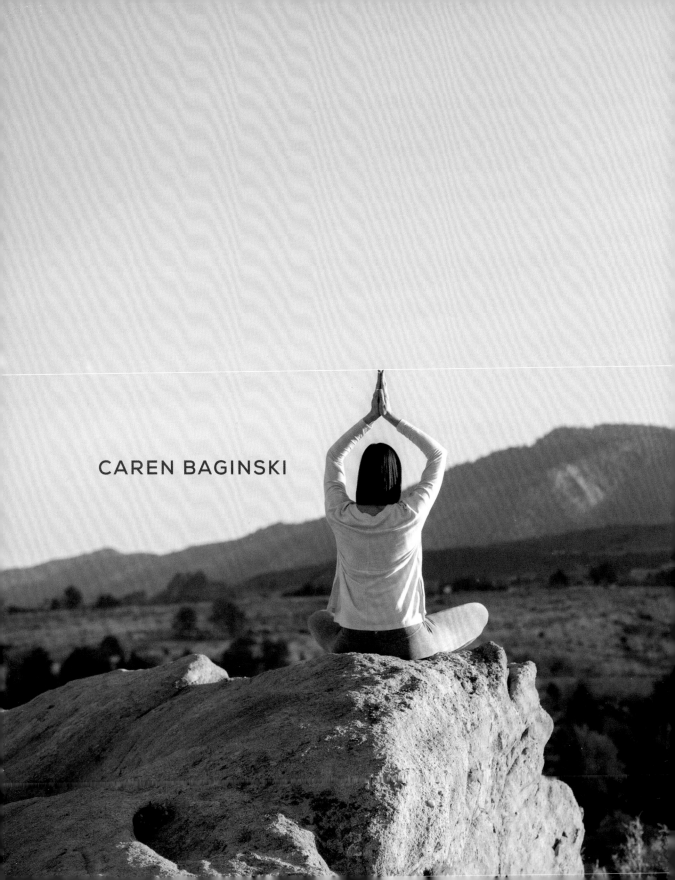

CAREN BAGINSKI

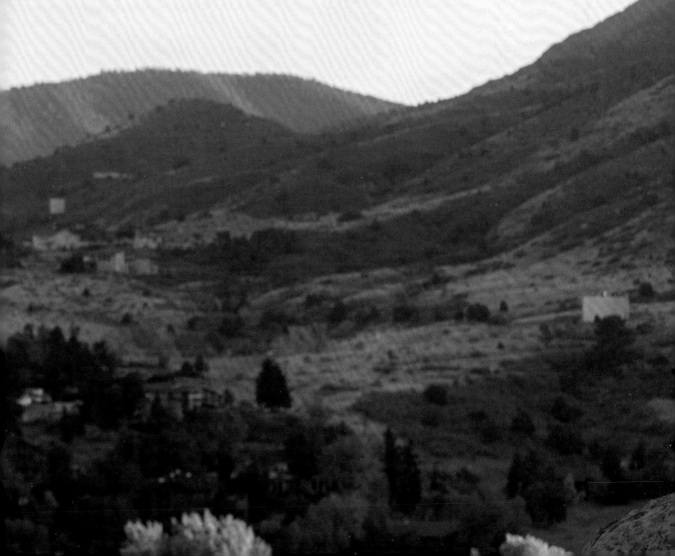

RELAX. RESTORE. RE-ENERGIZE.

Restorative yoga

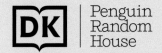

Publisher Mike Sanders
Senior Editor Brook Farling
Senior Designer Jessica Lee
Art Director William Thomas
Photographer Jimena Peck
Proofreader Monica Stone
Indexer Celia McCoy

First American Edition, 2020
Published in the United States by DK Publishing
DK, a Division of Penguin Random House LLC
6081 E. 82nd Street, Indianapolis, Indiana 46250

Published in the United States by Dorling Kindersley Limited

Note: This publication contains the opinions and ideas of its author(s). It is intended to provide helpful and informative material on the subject matter covered. It is sold with the understanding that the author(s) and publisher are not engaged in rendering professional services in the book. If the reader requires personal assistance or advice, a competent professional should be consulted. The author(s) and publisher specifically disclaim any responsibility for any liability, loss, or risk, personal or otherwise, which is incurred as a consequence, directly or indirectly, of the use and application of any of the contents of this book.

Trademarks: All terms mentioned in this book that are known to be or are suspected of being trademarks or service marks have been appropriately capitalized. Alpha Books, DK, and Penguin Random House LLC cannot attest to the accuracy of this information. Use of a term in this book should not be regarded as affecting the validity of any trademark or service mark.

A catalog record for this book is available from the Library of Congress.
ISBN 978-1-4654-9263-0
Library of Congress Catalog Number: 2019950631

DK books are available at special discounts when purchased in bulk for sales promotions,
premiums, fund-raising, or educational use. For details, contact
SpecialSales@dk.com

Printed and bound in China

Photo Credits: Dreamstime.com: Agnieszka Murphy / Redkoala; Dreamstime.com: Agnieszka Murphy
All other images © Dorling Kindersley Limited. For futher information see: www.dkimages.com

A WORLD OF IDEAS:
SEE ALL THERE IS TO KNOW

www.dk.com

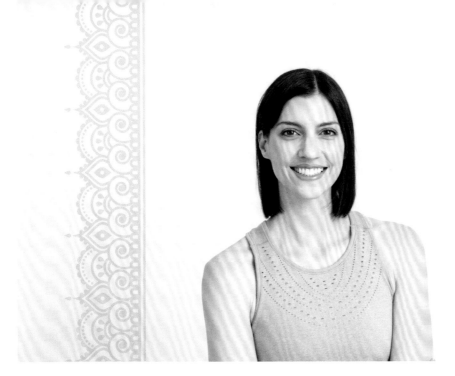

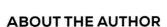

ACKNOWLEDGMENTS

Since I was 10, I've wanted to become an author. This book has truly been a dream come true that wouldn't have been possible without a tribe. First, to my husband, Evan, for his inexhaustible support and belief in me and my service in the world since the first day we met. To my dad, John, who taught me the importance of "stuff placing" that's so handy when teaching yoga, and my mom, Paula, my first spell checker, whose enthusiasm for my work is fuel. To Willow, whose tenacity and zest for life inspires me to never give up. To the pantheon of yoga teachers and realized beings (too many to name)—living and passed on—who have forever left their mark on my soul, in my yoga practice, and as a result, in my teaching. To my students and clients from around the world who trust me to be their guide and inspire me with their breakthroughs. And finally, all the gratitude to the publishing and photo shoot team who co-created this book with me, especially Brook, Jessica, William, Jimena, Tom, Nilesh, and Cindy, as well as Halfmoon for providing the props.

ABOUT THE AUTHOR

Caren Baginski, C-IAYT has been teaching yoga and meditation since 2009 and is the founder of *Being Enough*, a transformational process for gaining freedom from the negative inner critic and embodying deep rest and self-acceptance. Her YouTube channel has more than 1 million views and gives people from around the world permission to slow down, do less, and heal. In addition to restorative yoga, Caren is trained in Yoga Nidra and Vinyasa Yoga, and is a certified yoga therapist. A former journalist with a BSJ degree from Ohio University, Caren's writing has appeared in *Yoga Journal* and *Mantra Wellness Magazine*, among other publications in the home, health, and wellness industries. She lives in Denver, Colorado. Learn more at www.carenbaginski.com.

SPECIAL THANKS TO HALFMOON YOGA

The publisher would like to thank Halfmoon Yoga (shophalfmoon.com) for their generous contribution to the props used in the photos for this book.

Contents

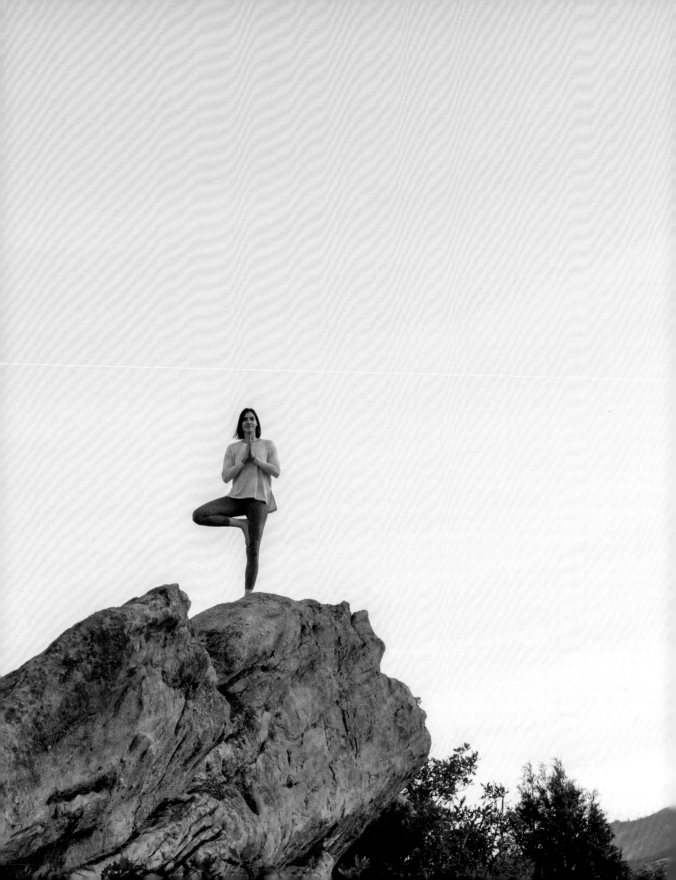

Introduction

What would your life be like if you took more time to rest?

Most of us feel like we can't afford to slow down and take a break. We face pressure in our jobs and at school to be more productive, make more money, or get better grades. We yearn for purpose or, upon finding that, seek continual self-improvement and growth because we still don't feel like we're enough just being exactly as we are.

Staying busy and rushing through life can have negative impacts on your health and well-being. In a world that doesn't slow down, we can either choose to slow down now or be forced to slow down later when our body develops illness, disease, or an injury.

Perhaps you're suffering right now, or you're looking for a path of prevention. Either way, it's an honor to welcome you to the practice of restorative yoga.

Practicing restorative yoga is a radical act of self-care and a declaration that your health and well-being matter more than checking off your to-do list. In this practice, you will experience firsthand that rest is a productive and necessary part of everyday living. Restorative yoga was a respite for me when I came out of depression, fractured my kneecap (which happened because I was rushing!), and it still helps me calm persistent back pain.

The balance, presence, and deep healing you desire will take root in the simple act of relaxing. This empowering practice will help you access the innate ability of your body to restore itself from stress. In as little as five minutes, you can decrease pain and muscle tension, elevate mood, increase immunity, enhance digestion, improve the quality of your sleep, boost learning and memory, and experience many more benefits.

Practicing restorative yoga is a commitment to presence—not running away or distracting oneself when thoughts or sensations arrive that aren't pleasant. It's easy to avoid or to distract ourselves from our minds and bodies; it's the commitment and willingness to stay present that brings transformation. Without even working your muscles, you will develop the strength and resilience to face whatever life brings.

In yoga, the mind and body are intertwined, so whatever you practice in the mind, the body becomes. The reverse is also true: What we consume through our senses alters the state of our minds. Restorative yoga is a mind-body approach to relaxation that gives us time and space to connect to a deeply peaceful, calm space within that is untouched by the weight of obligations, responsibilities, jobs, and relationships. By taking time to consciously relax, we can return to our natural stress-free state—over and over and over.

Whatever you're facing, may this book not only infuse your everyday life with lightness but also carry you through the dark.

Namaste.

Caren

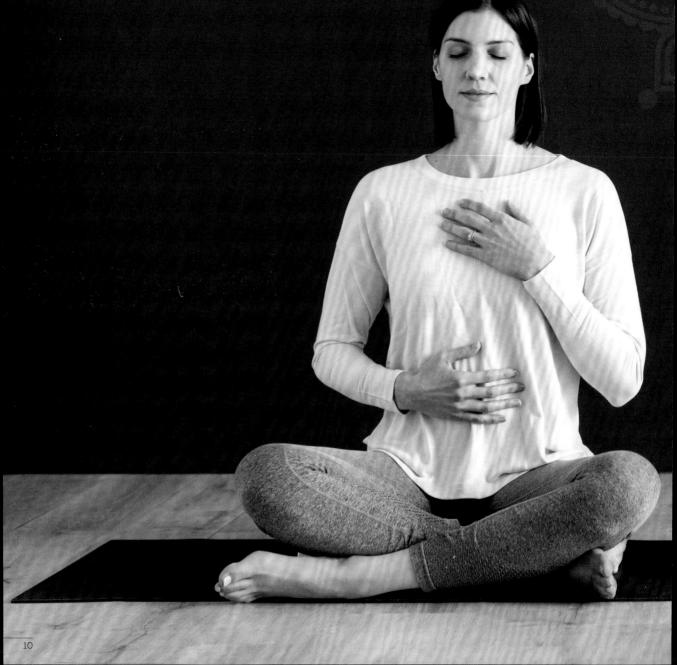

CHAPTER 1

Introduction

What is Restorative Yoga?

As you're about to discover, restorative yoga is a powerful mind-body-spirit practice that begins with a paradox: through the simple act of doing nothing, you can experience great shifts in your mental and emotional well-being, an expansion of vitality, smoother relationships, and increased creativity and productivity.

The restorative practice involves holding poses for longer periods of time while being completely supported by props so you can release all muscular effort and relax. As you do so, you remain awake and aware of your breath, and the subtle sensations that arise, whether physically, mentally, emotionally, or spiritually.

Doing less is more in restorative yoga, but how did we arrive at this realization?

A BRIEF HISTORY

Restorative yoga originated from the innovative teachings of B. K. S. Iyengar (1918-2014), the founder of Iyengar Yoga. A sickly child who struggled physically and mentally in his early life, Iyengar was invited as a teenager to live with his sister and brother-in-law, T. Krishnamacharya (1888–1989).

Iyengar was trained by Krishnamacharya, a highly influential yoga teacher and scholar who modernized Hatha Yoga as we know it today. Ashtanga and Vinyasa, the most popular yoga styles in the West, owe their roots to Krishnamacharya and to those he trained who spread his teachings worldwide.

Iyengar, however, took a different approach to teaching yoga. After improving his health through his yoga practice, the author of *Light on Life* began instructing independently and developed a method of therapeutic alignment and body awareness that included the use of props, such as ropes, walls, blocks, and blankets, to reduce strain and prevent injury in his students' bodies. His devotion to yoga as a pathway for personal transformation was passed along to his students, one of whom popularized restorative yoga as we know it today.

Judith Hanson Lasater, PhD PT, is another important contributor to the restorative movement. Lasater defined restorative yoga as a practice that utilizes props to create positions of comfort that help facilitate relaxation and health. Lasater met Iyengar in 1974 and studied with him for 25 years.

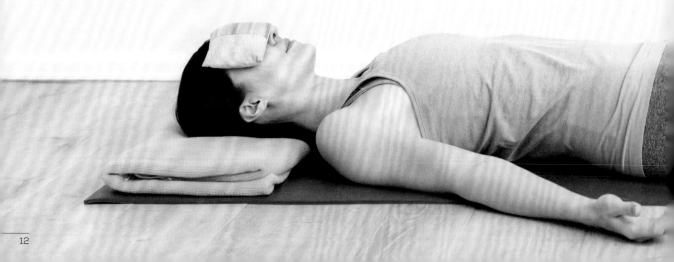

A MODERN PRACTICE WITH ANCIENT ROOTS

While restorative yoga may be relatively new, the science and philosophy of yoga is far more ancient. Yoga's exact origins are debated, but many Indian spiritual texts dating around the first millennium CE mention it, with the most well-known being the *Yoga Sutras of Patanjali*. In Sanskrit, the word *yoga* means "to yoke" or "to unite." Even though most people view yoga today as postures and breathing exercises, it began as a system to gain freedom from suffering and to remember your true nature. In essence, yoga is both the method and the goal of connecting with wholeness, presence, and deep peace.

Inspired by Iyengar, she and her daughter, Lizzie Lasater, train yoga teachers from around the world to teach this powerful practice. Although it is relatively new, restorative yoga has gained worldwide popularity with people who are entirely new to yoga, as well as experienced practitioners.

KEY PRINCIPLES OF A RESTORATIVE PRACTICE

There are four main principles that set a true restorative yoga practice apart. If you're following these guidelines, you'll know you're practicing restorative yoga.

- **The body is still.** Once the body is fully supported, you relax all effort and become still. In this way, restorative yoga is not about stretching or achieving—it's about being. Generally, you may hold poses from 3 to 20 minutes.
- **The practice space is dark or the eyes are covered.** Our natural circadian rhythms are programmed to wake us up with the dawn and wind us down with the sunset. Due to screen use and light pollution, however, many of us no longer live in sync with nature. Practicing in a dimly lit space or covering the eyes can help us to relax so we can restore that balance.
- **The practice space is quiet.** When exposed to consistently noisy environments (think car traffic and music-filled workspaces), your body's stress hormone levels can be chronically elevated. Give yourself the gift of silence, which has been found to be more relaxing to the brain than "relaxing" music.
- **The body is comfortably warm.** Just like a warm bath can ease tight muscles and reduce pain, staying comfortably warm with the help of clothing, blankets, or the thermostat can help deepen your body's relaxation response. And for many restorative yoga poses, you can keep your socks on!

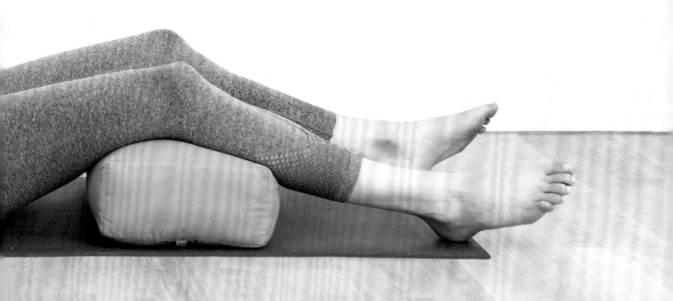

The Benefits of Restorative Yoga

When you embrace self-reflection, prioritize relaxation, and surrender to the process, you'll be amazed at the benefits you'll receive. Here are some ways in which restorative yoga can help you heal.

›› RESOLVES CHRONIC STRESS

Over time, the stress hormones cortisol, adrenaline, and norepinephrine can dampen the body's immunity, elimination and digestion functions, and sleep processes, creating disease in the body ranging from mood disturbances to reproductive difficulties. Restorative yoga facilitates the body in relaxing so that the adrenal glands can function properly, resetting balance in the autonomic nervous system from a "fight-flight-freeze" response to a "rest-and-digest" response.

›› SUPPORTS PHYSICAL AND MENTAL WELL-BEING

Now that you know how stress affects your body, what awaits when you practice restorative yoga is improved immunity, mood, and energy, as well as a calmer mind and more trust and purpose in your life path. The branch of the nervous system responsible for the "rest-and-digest" function is called the *parasympathetic nervous system*. Restorative yoga engages this branch, which slows respiration and heart rate, relaxes muscle tension, and lowers blood pressure. Research shows that this helps prevent stress-related diseases and improve the symptoms of anxiety and depression, as well as conditions like fibromyalgia, hypertension, and gastrointestinal distress.

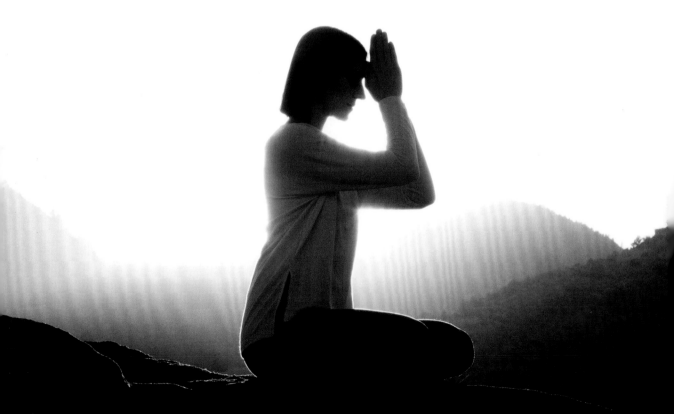

›› SOOTHES PERSISTENT PAIN

Persistent pain is not just "in your head" or isolated to structural damage in the body—it's a complete mind-body-emotion experience. When you feel pain, nerve pathways send signals to different areas of the brain—the limbic system (or emotional center) and the thalamus (to evaluate the pain). In this way, all physical pain sensations become linked to thoughts and emotions. Over time, accidents, trauma, illness, and stress can influence your body's protective responses and produce gripping muscles that can lead to postural shifts, which can then lead to shallow or held breathing patterns. The nervous system then becomes more sensitive to pain, creating persistent pain experiences such as low back or neck aches. Restorative yoga lessens these responses by calming the nervous system, assisting body posture alignment, and enhancing breathing to help your body relearn that it's safe.

›› HELPS ALLEVIATE HEADACHES

Restorative yoga poses, especially backbends, can help restore healthy spinal alignment in the neck, which can improve posture and reduce muscle tension to soothe or prevent headaches. Plus, using an eye pillow during practice does more than simply block light. When the eyelids receive pressure, this signals the vagus nerve, which is the tenth cranial nerve that runs down the brainstem to the belly, to turn on the relaxation response. Applying light pressure with an eye pillow to the center of the forehead can also be helpful. This space is the third-eye chakra, a subtle energy center relating to the ability to see beyond the sense of eyesight. Energetically, our relationship to our inner teacher resides here, and physiologically, tension headaches can express themselves around this area. For best results, seek dark, quiet spaces where you can relax.

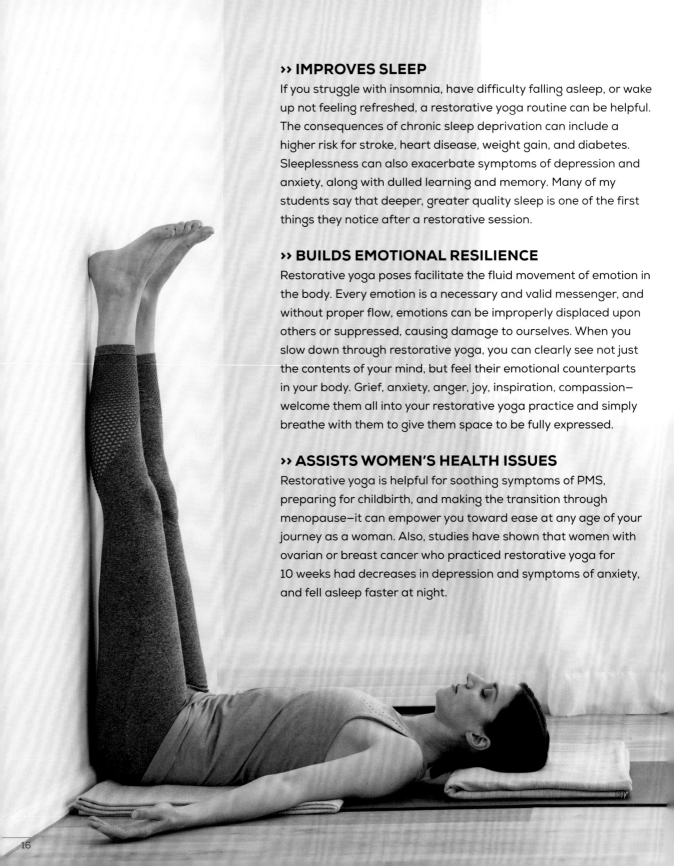

›› IMPROVES SLEEP

If you struggle with insomnia, have difficulty falling asleep, or wake up not feeling refreshed, a restorative yoga routine can be helpful. The consequences of chronic sleep deprivation can include a higher risk for stroke, heart disease, weight gain, and diabetes. Sleeplessness can also exacerbate symptoms of depression and anxiety, along with dulled learning and memory. Many of my students say that deeper, greater quality sleep is one of the first things they notice after a restorative session.

›› BUILDS EMOTIONAL RESILIENCE

Restorative yoga poses facilitate the fluid movement of emotion in the body. Every emotion is a necessary and valid messenger, and without proper flow, emotions can be improperly displaced upon others or suppressed, causing damage to ourselves. When you slow down through restorative yoga, you can clearly see not just the contents of your mind, but feel their emotional counterparts in your body. Grief, anxiety, anger, joy, inspiration, compassion—welcome them all into your restorative yoga practice and simply breathe with them to give them space to be fully expressed.

›› ASSISTS WOMEN'S HEALTH ISSUES

Restorative yoga is helpful for soothing symptoms of PMS, preparing for childbirth, and making the transition through menopause—it can empower you toward ease at any age of your journey as a woman. Also, studies have shown that women with ovarian or breast cancer who practiced restorative yoga for 10 weeks had decreases in depression and symptoms of anxiety, and fell asleep faster at night.

How to Transition from *Busy* to *Being*

When someone asks you how you are, have you ever responded with "I've been so busy"? *Busy* is an epidemic that keeps us feeling like we're at the mercy of our schedules, our relationships, and our work. *Busy* tells us we need to *have* more things in order to *do* what we really want, because only then will we *be* happy and fulfilled. This drive to search outside of ourselves for fulfillment will never satiate us, because there's always something more to achieve or acquire.

Restorative yoga flips this order. Through the practice, we establish *being* first. When you allow yourself to be exactly as you are, and through props you thoroughly support your body in this endeavor, you are restoring your senses so that you can then take clear action in the world. By taking time to consistently do less, you fuel yourself physically, mentally, emotionally, and spiritually to live a more fulfilling, healthier life where *busy* takes a backseat to the joy of *being*.

Here's a simple three-step yogic method from the *Yoga Sutras of Patanjali (Sutra 2.1)* to establish being so that you can invite greater well-being into your everyday life.

1. *Embrace self-reflection.* Throughout practice, remain present to your needs and adapt each pose so that it feels good in your body.

2. *Make a commitment to be consistent.* Create a routine or ritual of your practice, and stick with it. Shorter, consistent periods of practice are better than nothing at all, and will yield benefits sooner than if you wait for the perfect time to practice a longer sequence.

3. *Let go of expectations.* You might not feel relaxed every time you practice, and that's okay. Eventually, the mind, breath, and body will calm. Each time you practice, you are strengthening neural pathways that will help you return more quickly to the space of relaxation.

PRACTICING RESTORATIVE YOGA WHILE MENSTRUATING

When you're menstruating it's advised to keep your legs and hips level with, or lower than, your heart. In other words: you should avoid inversions. During inversions, the downward weight of the uterus may block blood flow, which could disrupt the natural menses flow. From a yogic perspective, this downward flow of energy is known as *apana*, and its function is to release and let go of what is no longer needed.

Preparing the Body for a Restorative Practice

While they're not necessary to fully enjoy a restorative practice, you may find it helpful to do some simple, active yoga postures to prepare your body for stillness. Because the emphasis in restorative yoga is not placed on stretching, these preparatory poses will increase your body's comfort and range of motion, and also expand your capacity for deeper, fuller breathing. Plus, if you find it difficult to be still and slow down, starting with gentle movement is helpful for discharging restless energy, making it possible for you to enjoy your practice more. These poses may be practiced as a sequence in the order shown or separately based on the tension you're experiencing in your body.

COW AND CAT POSE

Purpose: Warming up the spine
Duration: 10 breaths

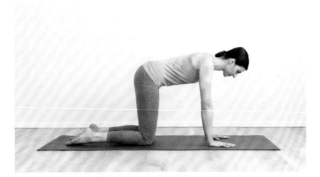

1. Begin in **Table Pose.** Place your hands, palms down, underneath your shoulders, and your knees under your hips. *(If your knees are uncomfortable, pad them with a blanket.)*

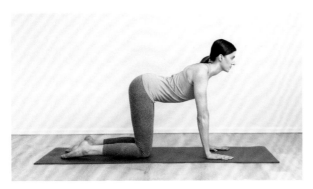

2. Come into **Cow Pose.** As you inhale, tilt your pelvis forward, then like a wave allow your lower, middle, and upper spine to descend toward the ground, letting the shoulder blades hug lightly together at the top of the inhale as you open the throat and gaze forward. *(If you have neck issues, keep the gaze down and your neck in line with the rest of your spine.)*

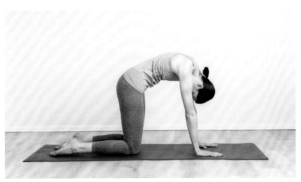

3. Transition into **Cat Pose.** As you exhale, relax the chin and neck downward, then round the upper, middle, and low spine toward the ceiling, feeling the navel lifting up as the tailbone tilts down toward the ground.

Continue smoothly between **Cow and Cat Pose** with full, expansive breath in the lungs for 10 rounds of breath, then arrive in a neutral spine and use one smooth breath to observe how the body feels.

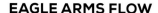

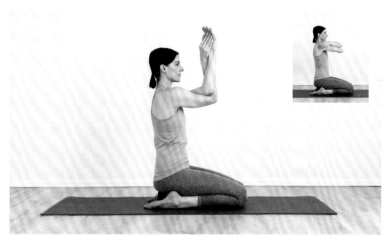

EAGLE ARMS FLOW

Purpose: Releasing tension from the shoulders and upper back
Duration: 5 breaths each side

1. Sit on a low block and extend both arms forward with palms down. Exhale and cross your right elbow underneath your left. Either touch your hands to the opposite shoulders (see inset) or lift the forearms to touch, optionally wrapping the right palm around the left. Lift your elbows to shoulder height, then lightly hug the shoulder blades in toward one another on the back.

2. Inhale and lift the shoulder blades and elbows comfortably high toward the ceiling, tipping the chin to look up.

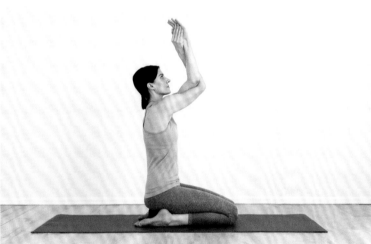

3. Exhale and lower the elbows down toward the chest, dropping the chin to your chest. Repeat steps 2 and 3 four more times, moving slowly with the breath.

Return the elbows to center, exhale, and unwrap the arms, releasing them by your sides. Roll the shoulders a couple times—up, back, down and forward—then repeat the pose with the left elbow underneath the right.

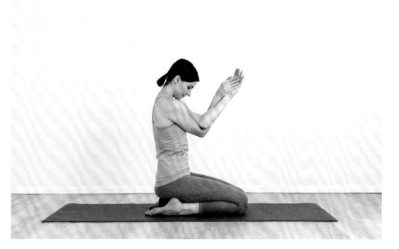

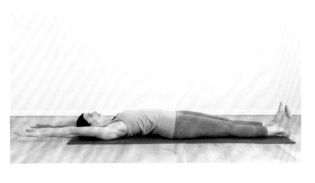

KNEES-TO-CHEST POSE FLOW

Purpose: Enhancing coordination and warming up the hips and shoulders
Duration: 20 breaths

1. Lying on your back, begin with your arms by your sides and legs outstretched. Inhale and raise both arms overhead, reaching from the armpit area, while simultaneously flexing the feet as if you were standing on the ground.

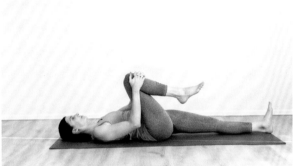

2. Exhale and lower your arms as you bend the right knee inward and take your hands to lightly clasp around the knee or shin. Inhale and stretch the right leg long and the arms overhead. Exhale and bend the left knee in as you bring the arms down to comfortably touch the left leg. Move back and forth, alternating legs with slow, steady, long breaths for 10 rounds. Take your time without rushing.

Once you've completed the rounds, relax your arms by your sides, widen your legs and relax the ankles, and rest for one more breath.

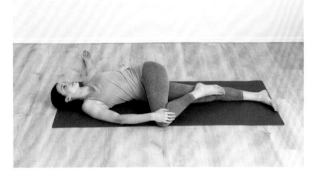

SUPINE SPINAL TWIST

Purpose: Rejuvenating the spine and stretching the chest
Duration: 5 breaths each side

1. Lying on your back, bring your left knee toward your chest, then cross it over the body to the right, using the right hand to support the left knee. At the same time, scoot your right hip directly underneath the left and extend your left arm away from your body.

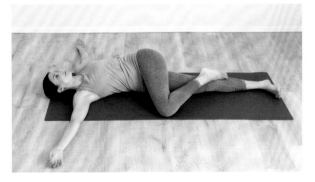

2. Open both arms wide to a *T* with your palms facing up. Stay in this position for five slow, deep breaths, then exhale, roll onto your back, and extend the left leg alongside the right. Integrate the experience with one round of breath before practicing the twist on the opposite side. *(If the low back is uncomfortable during the stretch, add a yoga block underneath the angled knee.)*

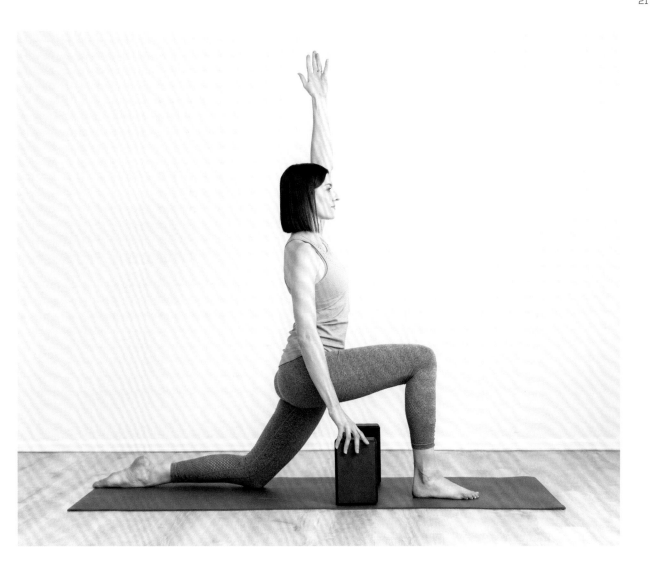

LOW LUNGE WITH BLOCKS

Purpose: Stretching the hip flexors and opening the chest for deeper breathing
Duration: 5 breaths each side

1. Begin in **Table Pose** with your hands stacked on two high blocks. *(If lunging on the ground is uncomfortable for your knee or not accessible, practice this same movement while standing and holding onto the back of a chair.)*

2. Step your right foot forward and between your hands to come into a low lunge, positioning your right ankle directly underneath your right knee. *(If your left knee is uncomfortable, pad it with a blanket.)*

3. Engage your inner thighs and inhale your torso upward, maintaining a level and square pelvis as you feel a stretch begin in your left leg. Place the fingertips of your right hand on the block for support or move your right hand to your right thigh for balance. Lift your left arm upward on the inhale, then stay for five full breaths, feeling the rib cage expand as you breathe.

4. Release your hands back to the blocks. Walk the blocks forward as you lean down toward the mat, carefully step your right leg back, and return to **Table Pose.** Practice **Cow and Cat Pose** three times, then repeat the movement on the opposite side.

Creating a Space for Your Practice

To further entice yourself to tune inward, it's important to design a practice space that creates the ideal conditions for relaxation. This place might be an entire room or just a simple corner in your home. No matter its size, when you attend to this area with intention it will become the container that supports you in self-exploration and slowing down. Here are some simple guidelines for creating your peaceful space.

CHOOSE A PRIVATE, CLEAN INDOOR SPACE

Your space can be carpeted or have hard floors, it all depends on your preferences for stability and how much softness you desire underneath your yoga mat. Ensure there's enough room to fully unroll your mat as well as ample room beyond the mat where you can easily move around and also keep props handy. When your space isn't in use, keep your mat, props, and timer arranged thoughtfully so they're always ready for practice, and vacuum or sweep the area regularly to keep it clean—maintaining a tidy, clean space can lead to a clear and uncluttered mind. Having an open wall nearby also is helpful for poses such as Legs Up the Wall.

When it's time to practice, set kind boundaries with housemates. Alert your family or roommates to when you're practicing so they know not to disturb you. Furry companions may not get the memo, so provide a space for them to rest nearby so they don't crawl on your yoga mat—even though they will. (I speak from experience!)

DIM THE LIGHTING

Close the blinds or curtains, turn off harsh overhead lights, and opt for shaded lamps or diffused light if you prefer some light while you practice. It may not be possible to shut out all light if you are practicing during the day, so keep an eye pillow or hand towel nearby to use as an eye covering. If it's not comfortable to cover your eyes, that's okay. It's more important that you feel safe so you can relax.

KEEP YOUR BODY WARM

Because the body's temperature drops when it lies in stillness, it's a good idea to always keep an extra blanket within reach for nearly every restorative pose. You can drape it over your whole body, or just a portion of yourself like your abdomen, feet, or hands. Avoid drafty areas, if possible, and keep fans or heaters blowing away from you. Socks may be worn in nearly all poses, except standing poses.

EMBRACE THE SILENCE

We live in a noisy world where sometimes it feels like everything and everyone is vying for our attention. Our minds are stimulated and inundated from the moment we awaken. Even during sleep, the sense of hearing never completely shuts off. The noisier the environment, the more reactive and distracted the mind. All of this to say: I encourage you to practice without music. However, if you live in a noisy environment or a bustling city, it may be helpful to use a white noise sound machine to drown out ambient distractions.

TURN OFF DEVICES

Consider using a simple kitchen or exercise timer that's not connected to the internet so that you can unplug during your practice. If you must use your phone as a timer, put it on airplane mode, turn off all notifications, and select a gentle, sweet-sounding chime that won't jolt you out of each pose. If you do fall asleep during a pose, no problem; the timer will guide you forward.

ADD BEAUTY AND COLOR

There are many ways to sweeten your practice space so that it becomes more likely that you'll make restorative yoga a regular ritual. What colors delight you and bring you peace? Are there quotes, intentions, or works of art that uplift you and bring you joy? Fill your space with a few meaningful items that inspire you to seek wellness.

KEEP A SELF-REFLECTION JOURNAL

Document your observations, insights, gratitudes, and feelings after each practice to track your progress and see the benefits firsthand. This can also be helpful for times when it feels like practicing is a struggle or not helping much. A journal will help you stay the course and celebrate your self-discoveries.

CONSIDER YOUR SPACE YOUR SANCTUARY

While there may be times when you choose to practice outside of your space, if you stay consistent with one location you'll be more likely to want to practice. Also, don't practice in your bed unless you're working through an injury or health condition and it's a necessity. Conscious deep rest and sleep are two different things, and maintaining this boundary is helpful for good sleep hygiene.

Choosing and Using Props

Props are an essential part of a restorative yoga practice. Without them, your body won't receive the necessary support to be completely comfortable and at rest. While you can substitute many things around your house for these props, here are my recommendations for a more enjoyable home practice. (Note that you can find these props online.)

BOLSTERS

If you invest in only one prop, make it the bolster. Bolsters vary in density, size, and shape, so finding one that fits your body is key for comfort. I recommend using a foam core or tightly packed cotton batting bolster that yields slightly under your body weight, while still providing enough firm support to be ramped on

blocks without collapsing. It's good to have both flat and round bolsters on hand as they serve different purposes in the practice, but if you're buying only one, choose the flat. (*Don't have it? Fold or roll thick, dense blankets to an approximate size of 5" x 10" x 24" (13 x 25 x 61cm) for a flat bolster, and 24" x 8" (61 x 20cm) for a round bolster.*)

BLOCKS

I recommend having at least two 9" x 6" x 4" (23 x 15 x 10cm) foam blocks on hand. Blocks also come in materials like cork and wood, but foam is lighter and offers firm yet gentle support, and it's also more comfortable than other materials. You can position the blocks in three ways: low, medium, and high.

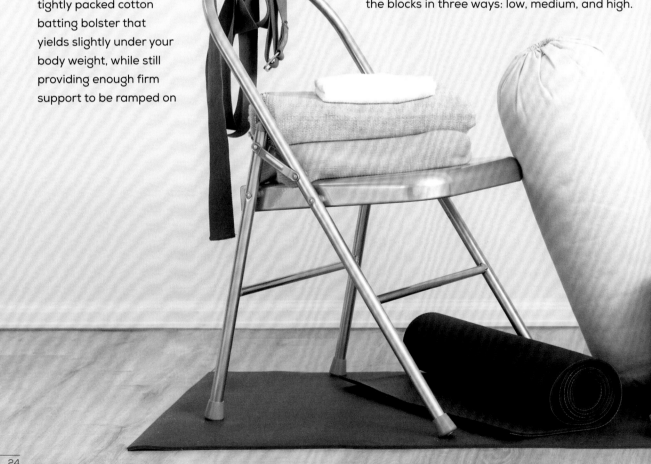

BLOCK HEIGHTS

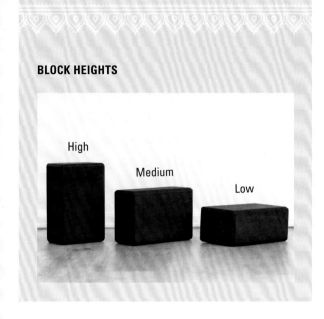

High

Medium

Low

STRAP

A soft yoga strap that measures 8' (2.4m) or 10' (3m) is a nice companion for practice. In many poses, it can be used to keep legs or arms in place so that they can completely relax. To loop a strap with a buckle, hold one end of the strap in each hand, thread the tail up through one half of the buckle, then back down through the other. Adjust the tightness by tugging on the long tail. (*Don't have it? Use a necktie or a belt.*)

CHAIR

Backless, armless folding yoga chairs work best for restorative yoga poses because they give your legs and feet ample room to practice the poses. (*Don't have it? Some poses can be improvised on couches or armless chairs that are low to the ground and have room to support the full length of your knees to your feet.*)

EYE PILLOW

To reduce light exposure and encourage deep relaxation, you may choose to cover your eyes with an eye pillow during practice. To enhance comfort and reduce pressure on the corneas, you should use only lightly filled eye pillows or a folded hand towel to cover the eyes, and remember to remove eyeglasses before using any eye covers. Eye pillows come in many varieties and shapes with different fabrics and fillings. Choose unscented if you have allergies or sensitivities to smells, or opt for one filled with lavender or other essential oils. Pick a fabric that's soft on your skin. Most pillows are filled with flax seeds or buckwheat hulls, which offer gentle weight to the eyes. (*Don't have it? Use a folded washcloth, which also is useful if an eye pillow creates too much pressure on your eyes.*)

HAND TOWEL

A folded 16" x 30" (40 x 75cm) hand towel is useful for elevating your head and wrapping around your eyes and ears to calm your senses.

BLANKETS

There are many ways to creatively use blankets, but here are the folds referenced throughout the poses in this book. Mexican blankets that measure 74" x 50" inches (188 x 127cm) are popularly used as props for restorative yoga, but there are other options if the acrylic fabric is irritating to your skin. If you prefer something softer and larger to cover your body, use a cotton blanket that's 60" x 80" (152 x 203cm).

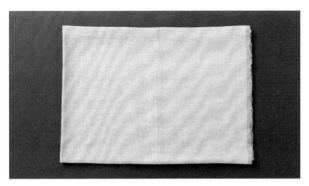

Basic fold
20"W x 28"L (51 x 71cm)

Open the blanket. Fold the two short sides together. From the new short side, repeat the fold. Repeat a third time. (This is the basic shape from which many other blankets folds are created.)

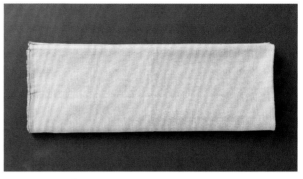

Rectangle fold
10"W x 30"L (25 x 76cm)

Fold the basic-fold blanket in half across its length so that it resembles a skinny rectangle.

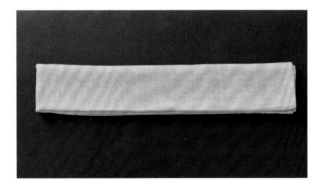

Long-rectangle fold
7"W x 41"L (18 x 104cm)

Starting from an open blanket, fold in half once from the long side. Again from the long side, fold in half. From the new short side, fold in half. Finally, from the long side, fold in half.

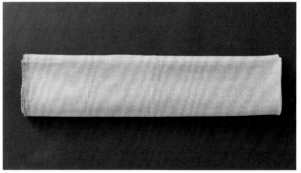

Double-rectangle fold
7"W x 30"L (18 x 76cm)

Begin with the basic-fold blanket. Fold about a third of each long end into the center, stacking one fold on top of the other.

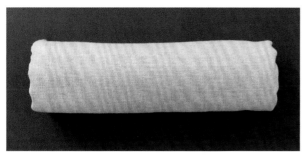

Rolled

4"W x 30"L (10 x 76cm)

Tightly roll up the shortest side of a basic-fold blanket.

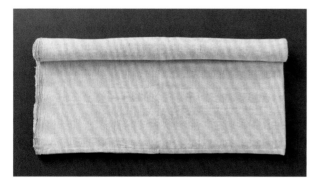

Half-rolled

9"W x 30"L (23 x 76cm)

Tightly roll the longest side of the basic-fold blanket only halfway, leaving some of the blanket unrolled.

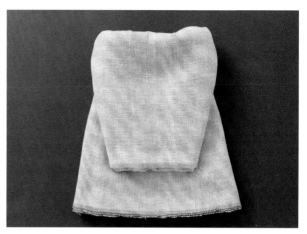

Headrest

12"W x 17"L (30 x 43cm)

Begin with a square-fold blanket. Take 2" (5cm) of the top fold and pull it back to reveal the bottom layer. Tuck the top layer's outer edges down and under to cradle each side of your head, then do the same for the bottom layer, tucking the outer edges down and under. Lie down on the blanket so that your head is in the middle and your shoulders are resting on the bottom fold with the edge of the top fold supporting the bony protrusion at the base of your skull. Finally, tuck the top-most corners under the skull to lift the forehead higher than the chin.

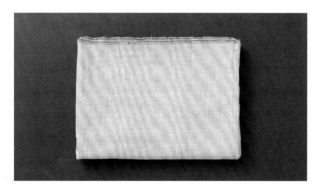

Square fold

15"W x 20"L (38 x 51cm)

From the basic fold, fold the short side once more to form a thicker yet smaller shape.

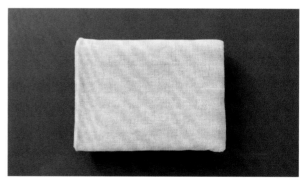

Double-square fold

10"W x 15"L (25 x 38cm)

Begin with a square-fold blanket. From the short side, fold in half.

Practicing Safely to Support Your Body

Before I give you a list of guidelines for practicing restorative yoga safely, there's another teacher you should be aware of who knows you better than anyone else and who will be your best mentor during this practice. That teacher is *you.*

Through the courageous act of taking time to do less, you have the opportunity to get to know yourself in a new way. Your inner teacher, or *observer,* is the part of you that remains unattached to the process and the results of your practice.

When we take time to become the observer of our life, rather than the doer, we finally have space to see ourselves as who we really are—beyond our age, physical limitations, the stories of our past, and our current moods. By cultivating deeper self-awareness, you can greet the higher Self that is untouched by struggle and suffering, and come to know yourself as free, peaceful, and limitless.

To embody this, it's important to check in when practicing restorative yoga, rather than checking out. According to yoga philosophy, we are multidimensional beings who have five subtle layers, called *koshas,* that we can bring into balance to remember our true nature. When you tap into these five aspects, you will discover that practicing safely is much more than simply "if my knee hurts, I come out of the pose."

A NOTE OF CAUTION BEFORE PRACTICING

You should always check with your healthcare provider before beginning a new movement routine, or if you are uncertain if a pose is safe for you. If you're still unsure, seek out the guidance of a trained restorative yoga teacher to ensure a restorative practice is right for you. Note that not all yoga teachers are trained specifically in the restorative style, so be sure to ask about the teacher's certifications before attending classes or workshops.

SAFE PRACTICE GUIDELINES

We all need support from others in addition to our inner teachers—after all, that's why you're reading this book! Here's are some practical guidelines for keeping your practice safe and enjoyable.

- As you begin a pose, ask yourself these questions: 1. Are my muscles relaxed? 2. Is my breath smooth? 3. Do I feel safe? 4. Do I think I'll be okay later? 5. Is it easy to smile?
- Approach each practice with a beginner's mindset: If you can't get comfortable in a pose, try the suggested adjustments or pose variations.
- Follow the "precautions" guidelines for each pose to ensure you are practicing in a safe and beneficial way.
- Make sure your head and neck are fully supported in every pose.
- Wait at least two hours after eating before you practice to allow your food to digest and to help you breathe easier.
- When practicing a pose with a chair, always be sure to place the chair securely on a sticky mat to keep it steady and immobile.
- Follow the recommended times for holding poses, but also trust and listen to your body if you feel you need to come out sooner or stay longer.
- Take ample time after your practice is complete to properly orient yourself back into the room and the outside world, particularly if you will be driving soon after practicing.
- Make sure to wear loose, comfortable clothing that doesn't restrict movement or breathing, and remove any jewelry from your wrists and neck.
- Remove eyeglasses and contact lenses prior to using eye covers that may create pressure on your eyes. Also, set eyeglasses aside when holding poses, especially if the head is against a prop.

LISTENING TO YOUR INNER TEACHER

Ask yourself the following questions for each kosha and use your answers as guideposts for a restorative practice that's led by your inner teacher.

PHYSICAL BODY

- Am I forcing myself into the pose and stretching, or am I properly supporting my body so I can feel more open and comfortable?
- Am I able to release tension from the crown of my head to the tips of my toes?

ENERGY BODY

- Is my breathing labored or shallow, or am I holding my breath, and can I adjust myself so that it is light, spacious, and free?
- Is the experience of my five senses pleasant in what I see, hear, smell, taste, and touch?

MENTAL AND EMOTIONAL BODY

- Am I suppressing emotions from arising or allowing them to flow freely, whether that's tears, a sigh, or even anger?
- Can I offer myself acceptance when my pose looks or feels different than how I expected it to?

WISDOM BODY

- Am I consumed by habitual thoughts and stories while in the pose, and can I kindly remind myself to come back to the present moment of what is happening now?
- Can I remain alert, not asleep, yet also deeply relaxed in my mind?

BLISS BODY

- Am I giving myself enough time in each pose to reach a space where I feel calm and peaceful?
- Am I transitioning slowly enough between poses to stay in a state of ease, rather than rushing my way from pose to pose?

Tips for Calming the Mind

Too often, our hectic pace of living and busy schedules hijack our capacity to be comfortable with slowing down and relaxing. Yet taking time to relax without additional stimuli is exactly what we need to restore and maintain our health so we can experience less stress and more enjoyment—even if the pace of our life doesn't slow.

You may have tried meditating before and thought that you were bad at it. The great news is that it's completely normal to feel like you can't "quiet" your mind when you try to relax. In fact, it's the brain's function to think. Even the most practiced yoga students sometimes have trouble quieting the mind.

I encourage you to drop all expectations of what your mind "should" be like when you practice and give yourself permission to accept yourself exactly as you are. You are not a failure if you find it difficult to relax—you are a human being who is taking steps to bring yourself back into balance. It's the steps that matter; the goal will come with consistent practice.

The gateway to calming your mind is through your senses. Our senses are always giving our mind feedback about the environment, so what you see (or don't see) and hear (or don't hear) has a direct effect on the state of your thoughts.

Here are a few suggestions for transforming your relationship with your mind as you practice restorative yoga.

COVER YOUR EYES AND EARS

In poses where you're lying on your back, you can apply an eye pillow or folded hand towel in different ways for a soothing effect on your body and mind. Here are a few ways you can use these props to increase your relaxation:

» Remove eyeglasses and place the covering directly over the eyes to seal off light. If you have an eye condition, be sure check with your healthcare provider to ensure it's okay to apply pressure to your eyes.

» Place a medium block just behind, but not touching, the top of your head. Drape the eye pillow lengthwise across the block and over the center of your eyebrows and scalp.

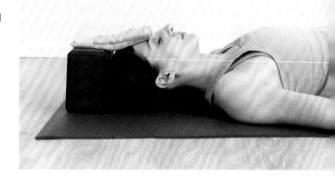

» Place the eye pillow horizontally so that it's resting on the forehead and just above the eyebrows. (This is a nice alternative to induce relaxation when it doesn't feel comfortable or isn't possible to close your eyes or place pressure on them.)

» Wrap your whole head in a folded hand towel to not only block light, but also sound. From the long side of the towel, fold it in half. When lying on your back, hold the short ends of the towel in your hands and hover the towel over your nose and forehead with the neatly folded edge toward your nose. Bring your hands down to the floor, lift the back of your head up slightly, and tuck the right side of the towel underneath your head. Keep holding both ends so that the towel is snug as you wrap the left edge on top of the right. Now lay your head down so the towel stays in place. If you are not lying down, you can drape the towel lightly over your head to conceal your eyes. (This is especially helpful when practicing side-lying poses or when it's not possible to put an eye pillow over your eyes.)

RELAX YOUR MUSCLES

To ease into deeper relaxation and release restlessness in your mind-body, practice the following body scan when you are lying in Basic Relaxation Pose. After you set up the pose, go through this progressive relaxation routine, a simple method of tightening and releasing muscle groups that has been shown to reduce pain, stress, and anxiety. Take a moment between each step to breathe fully and integrate the relaxation. When complete, rest for the remainder of time in the pose.

1. Inhale; squeeze and curl your toes and ankles tightly. Exhale; completely relax the feet.

2. Inhale, tense all the muscles of your legs, then exhale and release the weight of your legs into the ground and props.

3. Inhale, tighten your buttocks and outer hips, then exhale and release all grip and holding.

4. Inhale, make fists with your hands without strain, then exhale and completely relax your hands.

5. Inhale, squeeze the muscles of your arms and shoulders, then exhale and let go of the arms.

6. Inhale, purse the lips, scrunch the nose, wrinkle the corners of the eyes and eyebrows, then exhale and let all tension melt from the face.

7. Inhale, feel the whole body relaxing into the props and the ground, then exhale and let go from the head to the feet.

8. Breathe naturally and rest.

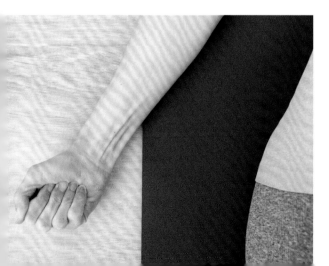

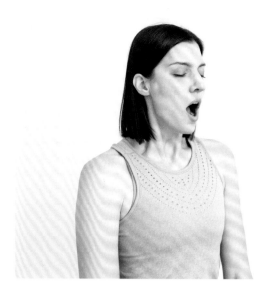

USE MINDFUL YAWNING

Yes, you read that right! You can shift yourself within minutes to a calm mental state through yawning. Not just for when you're tired, yawning activates the same structure in the brain (the precuneus within the parietal lobe) as yogic breathing and some meditation techniques. Studies show that yawning turns on a higher state of self-awareness and cognitive function while relaxing your muscles, increasing empathy and pleasure, improving coordination, and more. Many of us have been taught that yawning is rude or implies boredom. Toss that thinking out the window and yawn all you want during your restorative yoga practice. Here's how to do it:

1. Inhale deeply through the nose while opening your jaw wide.

2. Draw out a long exhale while making the sound of a sigh. If a true yawn doesn't happen right away, continue to "fake it" while pausing shortly between rounds. (It can be helpful to visualize yourself yawning and recall the memory of it while repeating steps 1 and 2 for at least five rounds.)

3. When your eyes start to water and you feel real yawns occurring, give yourself over to the experience for at least 10 more yawns. As the yawns subside, pay mindful attention to the quality of the mind, the breath, and the feeling in the entire body.

Breathing Techniques to Promote Relaxation

Restorative yoga gives us the opportunity to better understand a consistent friend we've had our entire lives: our breath. When we slow down and become still, we naturally become aware of our breathing, giving us insight into the state of our well-being. Modern science is now showing what the yogis knew ages ago: when restriction and friction in the breath is reduced, improved health is awakened.

Practicing breathing techniques during restorative poses is much more than just a fluid exchange of carbon dioxide and oxygen. By regulating and controlling the physical breath we can expand and maintain what's called *prana*. Prana is defined as the primary, smallest unit of indestructible energy that is the animating force of our life and the life of the universe. Through breathing techniques, you can remove blockages and smooth out the pranic pathways to create more balance and ease in the body, mind, and spirit.

Of course, you won't be able to see this happening—but you'll feel it. Most physiological functions of the body can't be controlled, but by taking advantage of changing the breath, you can shift your mood, calm the thoughts in your mind, pacify pain, improve sleep, and more.

The following techniques are used throughout the sequences in this book. If you want to experience a calmer state of mind, keep in mind four key attributes of the breath—quiet, steady, continuous, and prolonged—and invoke these qualities as you practice each technique.

EQUAL BREATHING

This foundational technique will help you create a calm rhythm with your breath so you can naturally deepen your breathing capacity—and your state of relaxation—without effort. To begin, empty your air with an exhale. With the spontaneous inhale through the nose, count of five, then exhale through the nose for another count to five. Use minimal effort to breathe smoothly in and out of the nose for a ratio of 5:5. Feel the abdomen, chest, and nose participating in this breath. If this count isn't quite possible yet, try counting 4:4 instead and work up to 5:5 over time.

LENGTHEN THE EXHALE

This technique is my go-to favorite for achieving a state of calm within minutes. After two minutes of performing this type of technique, stress levels are lowered and decision making can improve as a result of engagement of the vagus nerve and the transition to the body's "rest-and-digest" mode. Begin by exhaling through the nose, and inhale through the nose to a count of 4, then exhale through the nose to a count of 8. Keep an even pace with your counting and continuously breathe in and out completely from your abdomen and lungs. Practice for at least 10 rounds.

LONGER, SMOOTHER, SOFTER BREATHING

This breathing technique from Neil and Lisa Pearson of Pain Care U is indispensable if you are experiencing persistent physical pain. It will help you shift your relationship to the pain, even if it's chronic.

To begin, become aware of your breath moving in and out of your body. Breathe through your nose or mouth, whichever is more comfortable. Continue this for a few rounds, and establish longer breaths for 3 rounds without any greater effort, making both your inhale and exhale slightly longer. Continue this and then add a quality of smoothness to the breath.

Equal Breathing

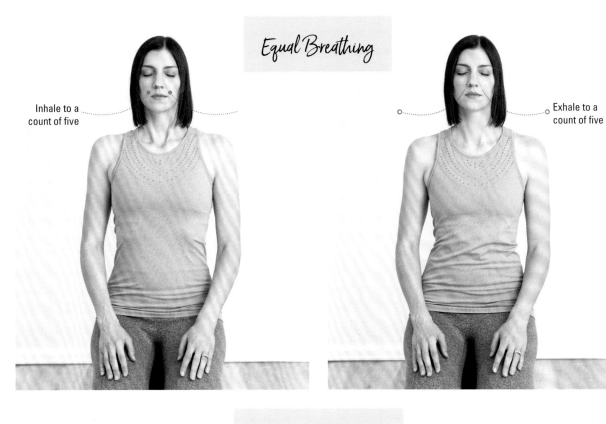

Inhale to a count of five

Exhale to a count of five

Lengthen the Exhale

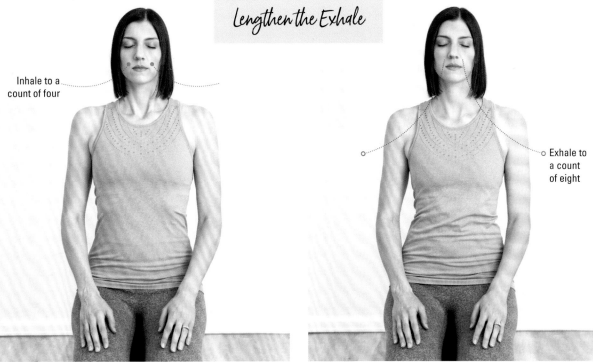

Inhale to a count of four

Exhale to a count of eight

Open Mouth Exhale

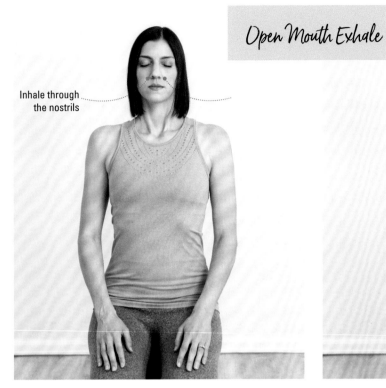

Inhale through the nostrils

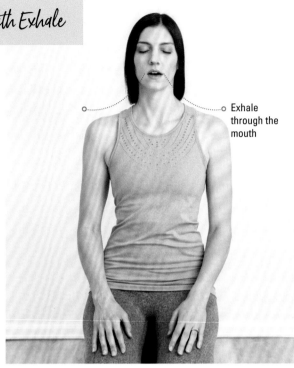

Exhale through the mouth

Alternate Nostril

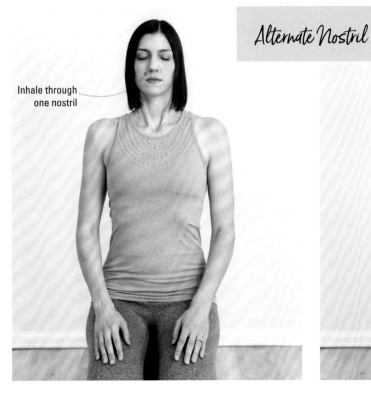

Inhale through one nostril

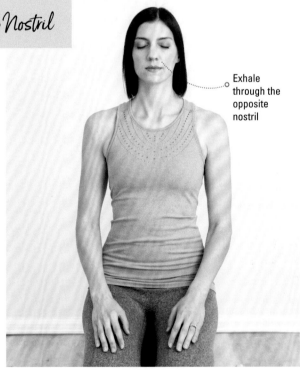

Exhale through the opposite nostril

Smooth out the transition of the inhale to the exhale and the transition of the exhale to the inhale for 3 rounds. Finally, add a feeling of softness by letting the breath glide easily without tightness for 3 rounds. Once you get the experience of all three attributes, practice them all at once for 10 rounds. As you practice this technique, sense the prana subtly moving into any areas of pain and tension with the intention of relaxing them.

OPEN MOUTH EXHALE WITH MANTRA

Breathing with a mantra is an effective way to stay present in the now and create space between thoughts. A mantra is a sound, word, group of words, or even a syllable that may be recited mentally or spoken aloud to invoke a specific energetic quality. Scientifically, repeating a mantra in the mind has been found to turn off activity in the default mode network: the part of our brain where we ruminate on self, others, the past, or the future.

To begin this technique, let the lips part slightly and relax the tongue. Inhale quietly through the nose, then exhale through the mouth and *imagine* whispering the word "relax" while emphasizing the vowel sounds ("reeeelaaax"). Exhale from the very back of your throat and extend the exhale. This helps prompt the deep relaxation response, plus you're also invoking the calming vibrational seed sounds of the throat (E) and solar plexus chakras (Ah)—subtle energy centers that live in the space of your breath. Practice 10 rounds, then close the lips and breathe naturally.

ALTERNATE NOSTRIL BREATHING VISUALIZATION

This classic breathing technique usually involves pressing one nostril closed with your fingers, but this variation allows you to visualize and practice the technique without movement, so that you can remain still in your pose. It will relax and balance the energy within the body, so you'll feel more centered and present.

To begin, imagine inhaling solely through the left nostril and following that air up to the point between the eyebrows, then imagine fluidly exhaling from the eyebrow center and down through the right nostril. Next imagine inhaling through the right nostril, then exhaling through the left. This is one complete round.

Continue the practice with longer, even, quiet breaths in and out through the nostrils, using the power of your imagination to "feel" the air moving up and down the nasal passages. Practice 10 rounds, then release the technique, breathe naturally, and observe how you feel.

BACK BREATHING

While we mainly think about and experience breathing in the front of our body, 60 percent of the lungs actually reside in the back half of our body. To access the three-dimensional capacity of your lungs, try this subtle technique. To start, perform the breath in three stages, then combine all three into one full breath that spreads across the entire back.

1. As you inhale, visualize the air expanding horizontally across the whole upper back so that each shoulder blade rises gently. As you exhale, empty the breath completely, while fully relaxing the upper back.

2. Inhale and visualize the air expanding horizontally across the middle of your back, beneath the shoulder blades and above the waist. Exhale and release the breath, relaxing the rib cage.

3. Inhale and visualize the air expanding horizontally across the low back and down to the hips, then exhale and relax all effort in the breath.

4. Release your abdomen fully. As you inhale, imagine the breath spreading horizontally across the upper back, the middle back, and the lower back. As you exhale, observe the spine feeling even longer from the neck to the seat. Continue for 10 breaths.

Poses to End Your Practice

If you ask experienced yoga practitioners and teachers, they'll say that the most important pose in yoga posture practice is *savasana*. Savasana is the final resting pose where you lie down on your back, become still, and integrate what has come before. In restorative yoga, this pose is called *Basic Relaxation Pose,* and it remains the most important pose of the practice and typically is held for 10-20 minutes. In fact, every sequence in this book ends with some variation of it. And don't despair if you find lying on the floor on your back uncomfortable—there are many varieties to explore here.

FOR EVEN DEEPER RELAXATION...

- Cover the entire body with a blanket and wear socks to keep warm.
- Place blankets underneath the wrists for slight elevation, then tuck the hands into the folds for warmth.
- Hold eye pillows in the palms of the hands to encourage heaviness and letting go in the hands.
- Add an eye pillow to the eyes or wrap the head with a hand towel to block out light.
- Ground yourself by placing a rolled blanket at the base of the wall and resting the soles of your feet on the blanket.

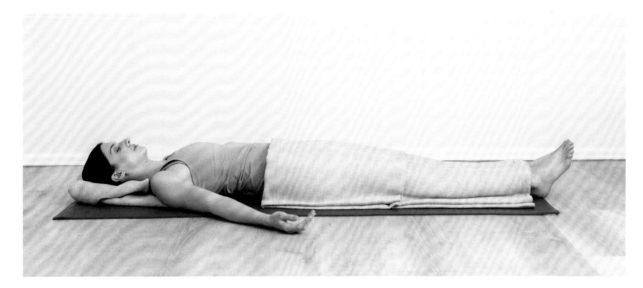

WRAPPED RELAXATION POSE

WHAT YOU NEED:
- Mat
- Blankets (1 headrest, 2 basic fold)
- Eye pillow (optional)

This variation is a balm for anxiety and will keep your body warm if you tend to get cool during practice.

Place the headrest blanket at the top end of the mat. Sit in the middle of the mat facing away from the headrest blanket. Extend your legs long. Take one basic-fold blanket and drape it lengthwise on top of the ankle creases and lower legs, with an even amount of blanket spilling off each side of your body. Firmly tuck the blanket underneath the outer legs and outer knee joints, then do the same with the second basic-fold blanket, allowing it up come up over the abdomen toward the low ribs. Lie back and extend the arms to a *V* with palms up.

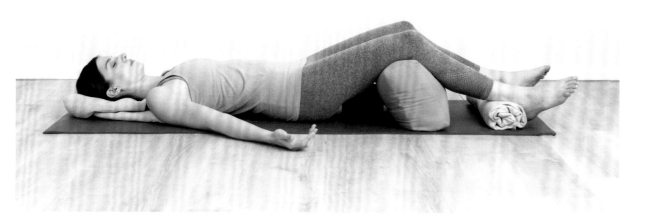

BASIC RELAXATION POSE

WHAT YOU NEED:

- Mat
- Blankets (1 headrest, 1 rolled)
- Round or flat bolster
- Block (optional)
- Eye pillow (optional)

Holding this pose for 20 minutes a day is a complete restorative practice in and of itself. If you're short on time, let this be your daily go-to "sequence."

Before you enter the pose, you'll need to determine the positioning of your legs and arms in Basic Relaxation Pose. Start by lying flat on your back on the mat with no props in place. Extend your legs long and place your arms by your sides. Rotate your legs inward from your hips, dipping your big toes in toward one another. If they touch, move the legs outward until the toes can no longer touch, then just relax the legs. Place both hands on your abdomen, with fingertips touching near the navel and bent elbows on the floor. Keeping the elbows in

position, open the forearms and hands outward and down to the floor, with palms facing up. *(If it's uncomfortable to rest with your palms facing up, turn your palms down and then soften your elbows.)* Take note of your leg and arm positions, returning to this once the props are in place.

To set up the props, arrange a headrest blanket at the top of the mat and position the bolster on the bottom third of the mat. Place the rolled blanket at the bottom of the mat to support your ankles. Sit in the middle of the mat and recline back over the props with your heels resting off the edge of the rolled blanket and the bolster supporting your knees, making sure your feet are extended to the proper width. Extend your arms wide into a *V* with your palms facing up or down, whichever is most comfortable. *(If your knees are not twice as high as your ankles, place the bolster on the long end and angle it at 45-degrees, then wedge a block underneath your thighs to support the bolster.)*

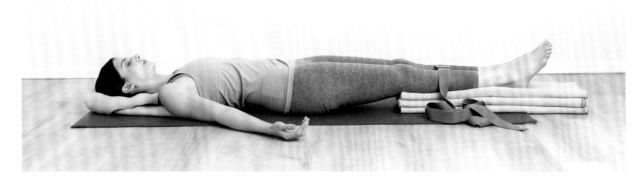

BASIC RELAXATION POSE WITH CALVES ELEVATED

WHAT YOU NEED:
- Mat
- Blankets (1 headrest, 3 rectangle fold)
- Looped strap
- Eye pillow (optional)

This variation provides relief for tired legs or lower back pain. It may also alleviate discomfort for women during menstruation.

Set the headrest blanket at the top end of the mat. Stack the rectangle-fold blankets lengthwise at the bottom end of the mat so that when you lie down the edges of the blankets support the backs of the knees, calves, and feet. To hold your legs in place, loop a strap around the middle of the calves, rotate each leg toward the other, and lightly cinch the strap. Lie back with your head in the headrest, then arrange your arms in a V with palms up.

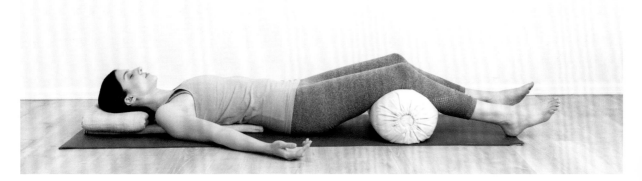

BASIC RELAXATION POSE WITH CHEST ELEVATED

WHAT YOU NEED:
- Mat
- Blankets (2 rectangle fold)
- Round bolster
- Eye pillow (optional)

This subtle variation assists with deeper and more effortless breathing by supporting the spine with a blanket.

Place a rectangle-fold blanket lengthwise along the top third of the mat, then place the second rectangle blanket, folded in half from the short end, at the top of the mat. Place the bolster widthwise on the bottom third of the mat. Sit with your hips against the bottom edge of the long blanket and your knees placed over the bolster. Recline until your head is supported, then extend your arms to a V with palms up.

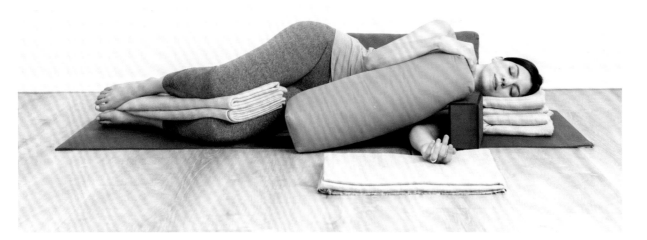

SIDE-LYING RELAXATION POSE

WHAT YOU NEED:

- Mat
- Blankets (2 double-square fold, 3 basic fold, 2 rectangle fold)
- Flat bolsters (1–2)
- Block
- Folded hand towel (optional)

If lying on your back feels unsafe or you experience overwhelm, worry, or fatigue, try this variation that sets you up to lie on your left side and also helps aid in digestion. Note that women who are more than three-months pregnant should opt for this pose to end their practice because the position keeps the pressure of the baby off the inferior vena cava, allowing for better blood circulation.

To start, set up the mat so your back will be against a wall, or position a flat bolster on its long side along the back edge of the mat. Stack two basic-fold blankets lengthwise down the middle of the mat. (You may prefer to add more blankets for extra padding if you're practicing on a hard floor.) Stack the two double-square–fold blankets at the

top end of the mat, then stack the two rectangle-fold blankets at the bottom end of the mat. In the middle and off the right side of the mat, ramp the flat bolster up a medium block and toward the top end of the mat. Set the basic-fold blanket on the floor and next to the ramp.

Sit on your left hip on the blankets and in between the bolsters, facing the bolster ramp. Place the rectangle-fold stack between your knees and ankles so that your feet are fully supported and your knees are at 45-degree angles. As you lie down, let the back bolster meet your hips and upper back, and rest your head on the square-fold blankets. (Your head and neck are supported so your chin can drop slightly downward and toward the heart.)

Reach your left arm underneath the ramp and place your wrist on the basic-fold blanket. Let your left shoulder blade be held by the floor. Place the hand towel over your head if desired. Drape your right arm over the top of the front bolster until the shoulder joint feels fully supported.

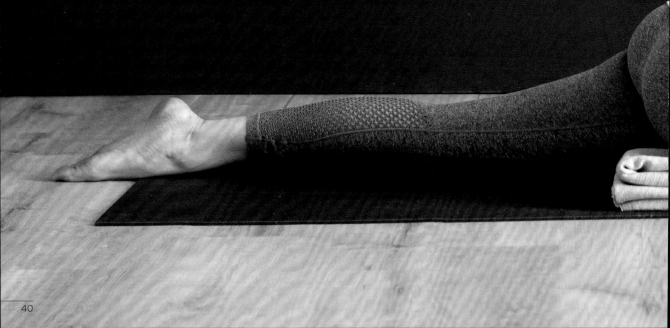

CHAPTER 2
Forward Bend Poses

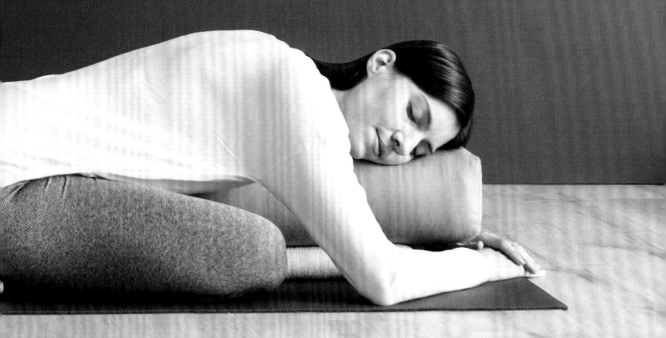

Supported Downward-Facing Dog

RECOMMENDED TIME // 1 MINUTE

This common yoga posture gets a restorative makeover with the addition of a block at the head. You may experience a deeper sense of grounding from this new perspective, as well as reduced tension in the legs, upper back, head, and neck.

WHAT YOU NEED
- Mat
- Block

PRECAUTIONS
Not recommended if you have a cold or sinus infection, eye issues, a hiatal hernia, uncontrolled hypertension, or osteoporosis. Follow the Safe Practice Guidelines (p. 28) for acute sciatica or injured hamstrings.

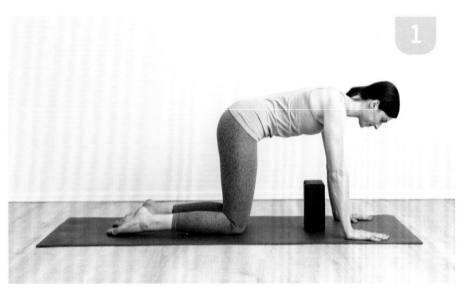

1 Place a high block in the middle of, and toward, the upper third of the mat. Start in Table with your hands and knees flat on the floor, and the block positioned directly under your chest. Widen your hands toward the outer edges of the mat while gently spreading your fingers and keeping the middle fingers pointing forward.

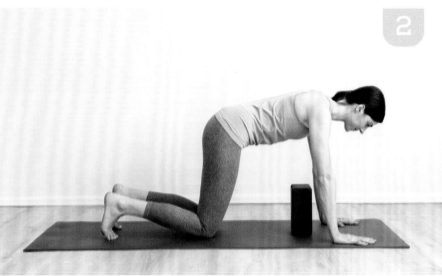

2 Walk your knees a few inches back from your hips while tucking your toes under.

EXPERIENCE THE POSE
Breathe smoothly and slowly, allowing the breath to inhabit your entire torso. There is no goal to stretch or deepen your flexibility, just think of becoming less active and holding with ease.

Maintain gentle curve in spine

Block should touch just above forehead

Lightly press into the knuckles of your hands and shift some weight to the index fingers and thumbs. At the same time, rotate your upper arms outward and press your shoulder blades inward and down. Exhale and lift from your navel and low belly to push your hips upward while tucking your chin and lowering your head until your forehead is resting easily on the block. Allow your heels to drop naturally to the floor. If needed, adjust the block height so that your head is resting with just moderate weight on the block. *(If you experience discomfort in your legs or back, try bending your knees slightly or widening your legs.)*

TRANSITION OUT: Exhaling, bend your knees and lower them down to the floor. Uncurl your toes and sit back on your heels or take a cross-legged seat. Notice the effects of the pose on your body and breath.

Half-Dog at Wall

RECOMMENDED TIME // 1 MINUTE

Awaken steadiness and stability in your whole body with just your mat and the wall. Turn to this pose for a boost in breathing or as a pick-me-up in the middle of the day.

WHAT YOU NEED
- Mat
- Wall

PRECAUTIONS
Not recommended if you have a cold or sinus infection. Follow the Safe Practice Guidelines (pg. 28) for acute sciatica or injured hamstrings.

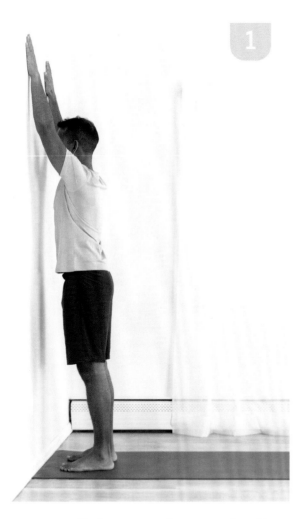

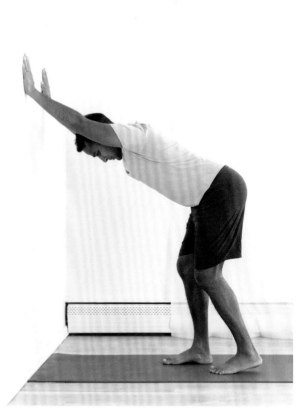

Find an open wall space and position the mat on the floor so that it's perpendicular to the wall. Stand, facing the wall, and place your palms flat against the wall, with your arms fully extended overhead.

Exhale and slowly slide your palms down the wall as you begin walking your feet back and away from the wall. Notice the backs of your legs lengthening as your palms stay anchored on the wall.

EXPERIENCE THE POSE
Begin with full, smooth breaths into the entire rib cage, expanding and emptying the breath throughout the front, back, and sides. Relax the jaw as you hold the pose.

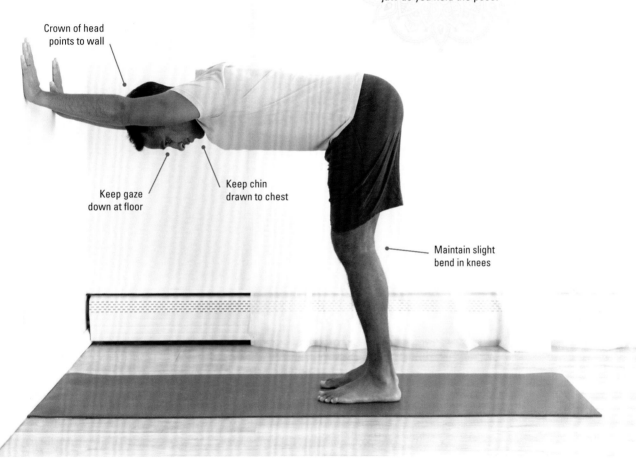

Crown of head points to wall

Keep gaze down at floor

Keep chin drawn to chest

Maintain slight bend in knees

Pause and hold when your upper body is perpendicular to the wall.

TRANSITION OUT: Release your hands from the wall and place them on your hips. Inhale, contract your thigh and calf muscles, and slowly rise to standing by lengthening the whole spine while avoiding rolling up.

Supported Child's Pose

RECOMMENDED TIME // 3–5 MINUTES

This calming position is as much a balm for a busy mind as it is an opening for the back muscles. To soothe your abdomen, it's important to substantially build the props underneath your torso until you feel completely held.

WHAT YOU NEED
- Mat
- Blankets (2)
  » 1 basic fold
  » 1 rectangle fold
- Flat bolster

PRECAUTIONS
Not recommended if you have a knee injury, or experience numbness or radiating leg pain while in the pose. Do not practice if you are more than three months pregnant.

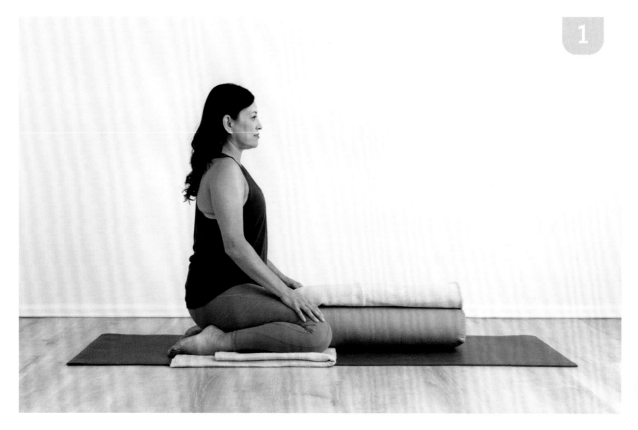

1

Place a basic-fold blanket widthwise across the middle of the mat, with the top fold supporting just underneath the ankle. Place the bolster lengthwise in the middle of the mat and above the blanket, and stack at least one rectangle-fold blanket on top of the bolster. Kneel on the blanket at the bolster's edge, widening your knees to each side, then bring your feet closer together and sit back on your heels. *(If you experience knee discomfort while in this pose, practice the variation with chairs or a ramped bolster instead.)*

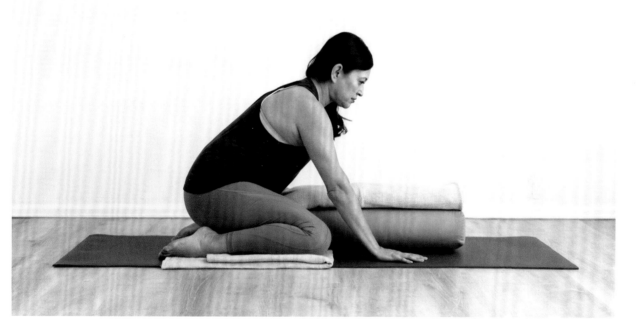

Inhale and feel your spine lengthening from your seat through the top of your head, then exhale and walk your hands forward to begin lowering your upper body down to the bolster. *(If there is still space between your abdomen and the props when you arrive at the bolster, add another rectangle-fold blanket until the whole front of the body can relax without effort.)*

Become aware of your soft
breath as the body settles. Give
yourself permission to make any
necessary adjustments to your legs or
feet so you may fully relax. Halfway
through the hold, you can switch
the head to lay on the opposite
cheek, if it's comfortable.

Hips are level
with shoulders

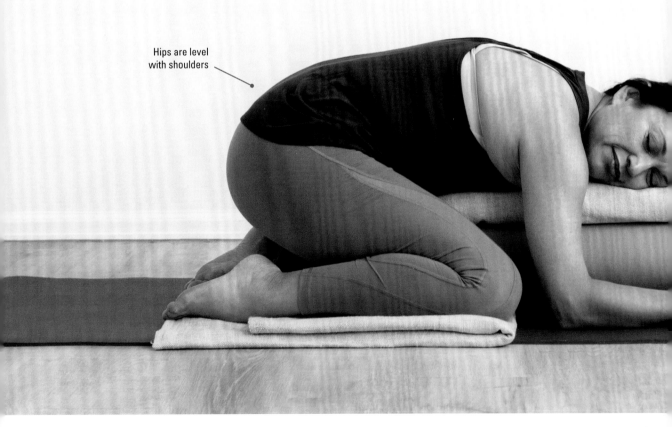

3

Turn one cheek to rest on the props and close your eyes, if it's comfortable. You can reach your forearms forward or extend them back toward your feet—experiment and settle with what feels most pleasant. Your palms can be facing up, down, or inward toward the body. Your neck should be completely relaxed while your shoulder blades melt open and apart.

TRANSITION OUT: Turn your forehead to face the bolster first, then, with your hands by your sides, exhale and use just enough effort to push into the floor and slowly lift the torso. Walk the knees back to Table with your upper body hovering over the bolster. Extend one leg straight back at a time, with toes tucked into the floor, and take three deep breaths on each side to allow circulation to flow through the knees and ankles.

Variation

To accommodate discomfort in knees and ankles, practice this variation. Add two blocks underneath the bolster, a rolled blanket between your legs, and a half-rolled blanket underneath the ankles. Slide your arms between the blocks and rest the forearms on the floor.

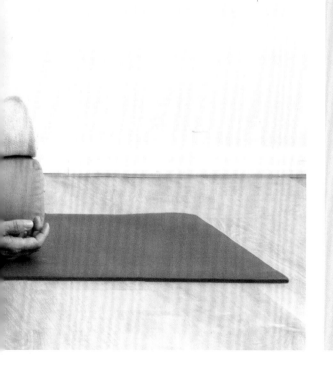

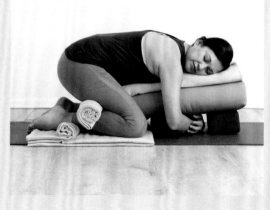

Supported Child's Pose
with chairs

RECOMMENDED TIME // 3-5 MINUTES

This gentler variation of Supported Child's Pose is beneficial when recovering from a knee or hip injury, or simply when practicing on the floor is too cumbersome. Allow the chairs to fully support your body in this gentle forward bend that will help your mind reach a more peaceful state.

WHAT YOU NEED
- Mat
- Blankets (1–2)
  » 1-2 rectangle fold
- Flat bolster
- Block
- Strap
- Chairs (2)

PRECAUTIONS
Do not practice if you are more than three months pregnant.

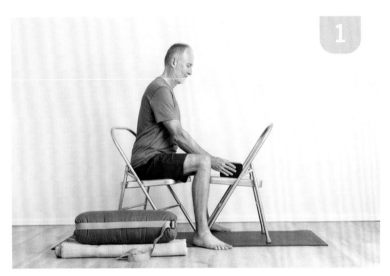

Tightly secure the yoga strap around the circumference of the bolster. Position the chairs facing one another on the mat, with one chair turned at an angle so that the corner of the seat is pointing to the center of the other chair. Sit in the angled chair, then straddle the other chair with your legs, keeping your feet flat on the floor. Place a low block in the center of the chair. (If your feet do not easily touch the floor, you can place blocks underneath them.)

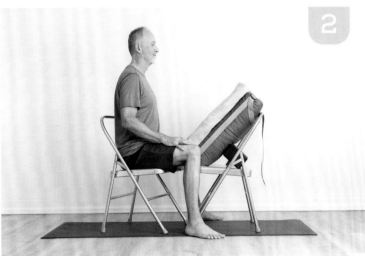

Set one end of the bolster on the chair and ramp it up the chair, adjusting the angle of the block as needed to support the bolster. Place the rectangle-fold blanket over the bolster.

3

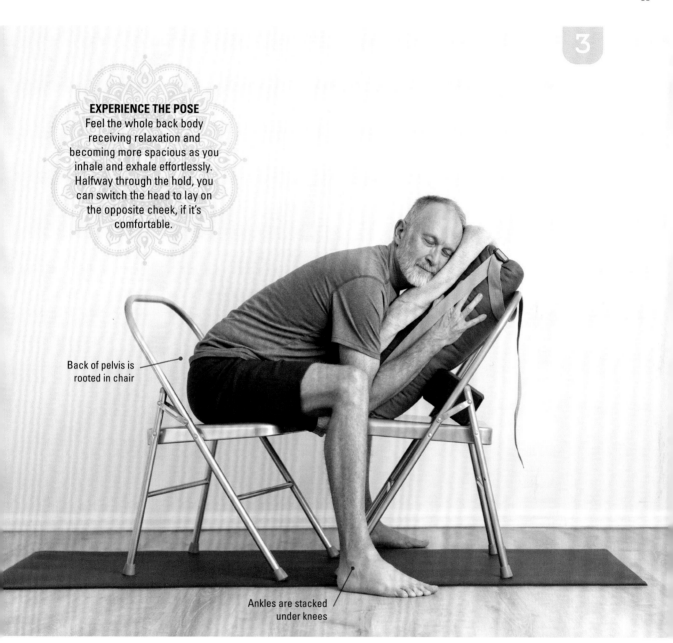

EXPERIENCE THE POSE
Feel the whole back body receiving relaxation and becoming more spacious as you inhale and exhale effortlessly. Halfway through the hold, you can switch the head to lay on the opposite cheek, if it's comfortable.

Back of pelvis is rooted in chair

Ankles are stacked under knees

Lean forward and onto the bolster, turning one cheek to the blanket, until your upper body is fully supported and your spine is evenly bending forward. Slide your hands underneath the strap and allow your elbows to relax completely. Close your eyes, if it's comfortable. *(If you need more support under your abdomen, add an additional rectangle-fold blanket on top of the bolster.)*

TRANSITION OUT: Release your hands toward the chair in front of you. Press gently into your palms, exhale, and lift your upper body upright to a seated position.

Supported Child's Pose
with ramped bolster

RECOMMENDED TIME // 3-5 MINUTES

If tight leg muscles, tension in the knees, or ankle stiffness aren't resolved with Supported Child's Pose, try this variation instead. While the setup is more involved, it may help with lower leg pain, and the resulting feelings of stability and tranquility make it well worth the effort.

WHAT YOU NEED
- Mat
- Blankets (2)
  » 1 basic fold
  » 1 rectangle fold
- Flat bolster
- Blocks (3)
- Strap

PRECAUTIONS
Not recommended if you have a knee injury, or experience numbness or radiating leg pain while in the pose. Do not practice if you are more than three months pregnant.

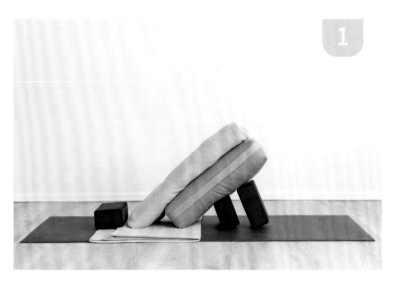

1 Snugly secure the strap lengthwise around the circumference of the bolster. Place the basic-fold blanket widthwise across the middle of the mat with the top edge of the blanket folded just short of the bottom edge. Position the blocks, one medium and one high, in front of the blanket, then ramp the bolster on top of the blocks. Place the rectangle-fold blanket lengthwise on top of the bolster. Set the low block widthwise at the base of the bolster ramp.

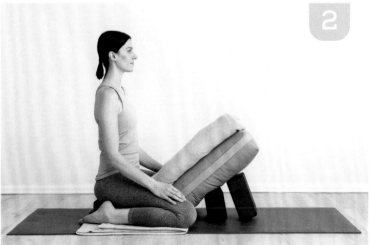

2 Straddle the base of the bolster and sit back on the block with your hands resting on your thighs and your ankles positioned just above the top fold of the blanket. Inhale and grow tall through your spine, then exhale as you begin to lower your upper body down to the bolster. (If the block is uncomfortable, sit on a double-square-fold blanket instead.)

3

Turn one cheek to the side as you arrive at the bolster. Bend your elbows and snug your hands in between the strap and bolster, with your palms facing in.

TRANSITION OUT: Exhale, slip your hands out of the strap and down to the floor, and sit up slowly. Move the bolster ramp and blocks off to the side of the mat. Walk the hands forward to Table, lifting your hips above your knees. One at a time, extend a leg straight back, toes tucked into the floor, and take three deep breaths on each side to allow circulation to flow through the knees and ankles.

EXPERIENCE THE POSE
Prompt yourself with an exhale to let go of any residual tension or tightness in your shoulders, back, hips, and feet, then just breathe naturally. Halfway through the hold, you can switch your head position to the opposite cheek, if it's comfortable.

Arms are effortlessly held in place and elbows are completely relaxed

Variation

If you'd prefer not to restrict your arms under a strap or require more height in your hips, try this variation. Place one end of the flat bolster on top of a round bolster, then stack the blocks under the opposite end of the flat bolster for support. Set two rolled blankets at your knees as armrests. Straddle the round bolster with your knees positioned wider than your feet.

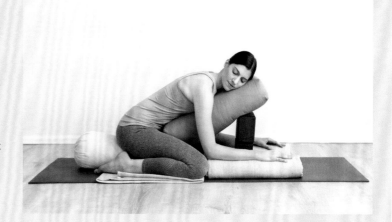

Surfboard

RECOMMENDED TIME // 5 MINUTES

This belly-down pose is a helpful alternative when bending the knees in Supported Child's Pose isn't comfortable or possible. It's also deeply calming for the mind and nourishing for the digestive system because the abdomen is pressed into a bolster.

WHAT YOU NEED
- Mat
- Blankets (2)
  » 1 rolled
  » 1 square fold
- Flat bolster
- Rolled hand towel

PRECAUTIONS
Do not practice until at least 2 hours after eating or if you are more than three months pregnant. Consult with a healthcare professional about osteoporosis, a hiatal hernia, or surgery in the chest or abdomen.

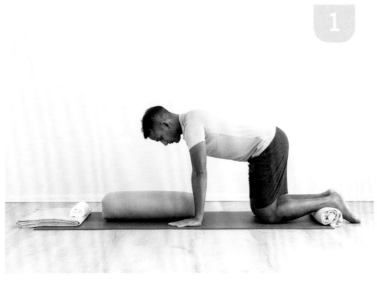

1 Place the rolled blanket across the bottom end of the mat. Position the bolster lengthwise in the middle, and toward the top end of the mat. Place the square-fold blanket at the top of the mat and a few inches from the bolster. Set the rolled hand towel on top of the blanket. Begin in Table with your ankles draped over the rolled blanket and hands at the base of the bolster.

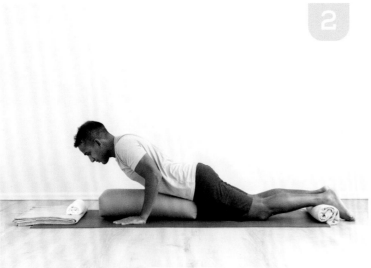

2 Begin walking your hands forward while lowering your body down until the edge of your pubic bone arrives on the bottom edge of the bolster and your belly is resting on the bolster.

3

EXPERIENCE THE POSE
Your eyes have nothing to gaze at here but the blanket. Perhaps close them and draw your senses further into your inner experience. Practice Back Breathing or simply enjoy the heaviness of your entire body giving in to gravity.

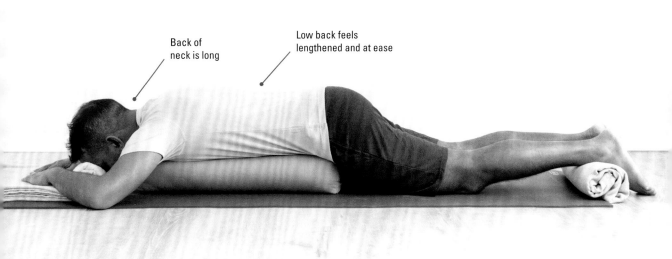

Back of neck is long

Low back feels lengthened and at ease

Continue to lower until your forehead is resting on the hand towel, then slide your forearms forward, bending the elbows outward, until your palms are flat on the square-fold blanket. If necessary, adjust the height of the blanket and hand towel so the nose is lifted above the floor and the chin can dip inward and slightly toward the throat.

TRANSITION OUT: Bend your elbows to return your palms to a position by your shoulders. On an exhale, gently engage your abdomen and press into your knees and hands to walk back up to Table.

Supported Seated Bound Angle

RECOMMENDED TIME // 3-5 MINUTES

Similar to Supported Seated Angle, this pose swaps extended legs for bent knees and also brings together the soles of the feet. This calming position is a tonic for tight hips and helps carry the focus inward.

WHAT YOU NEED
- Mat
- Blankets (5–6)
  » 1 square fold
  » 2 rolled
  » 1–2 rectangle fold
  » 1 double-square fold
- Flat bolster

PRECAUTIONS
Do not practice if you have a hiatal hernia. Follow the Safe Practice Guidelines (p. 28) if you have sacroiliac or knee pain. If more than three months pregnant, try the variation.

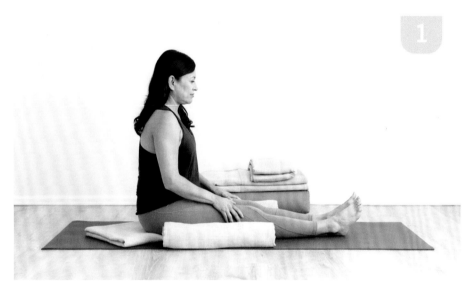

1 Place the square-fold blanket across the middle of one end of the mat, with a neatly folded corner pointing up the middle, and place the two rolled blankets at the sides of the mat. Stack the 1–2 rectangle-fold blankets on top of the bolster, then place the double-square-fold blanket at the top end of the bolster. Sit on the edge of the square-fold blanket and extend your legs out in front of you.

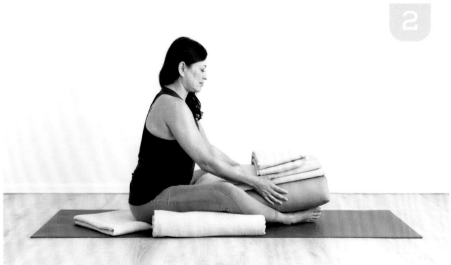

2 Bend at the knees to pull your feet in toward your groin while simultaneously dropping your knees toward the ground and bringing the soles of your feet together. Pull the rolled blankets in and underneath the upper thigh and midcalf regions to support the knees. Ramp the bolster in front of you and on top of your ankles.

3

Inhale, lengthen your spine upward, then exhale and reach your upper body forward as you lower down to the support in front of you. Rest your arms comfortably on either side of the bolster, relaxing your hands on the mat. Rest the eyebrow center to the double-square-fold blanket and tuck your chin slightly toward your chest to elongate the neck. Close your eyes, if it's comfortable.

TRANSITION OUT: Exhale and push your palms gently into the floor to lift your torso upward without rolling your spine. Remove the props from your legs. Support the outer knees with your hands and bring the legs together. Extend the legs and relax for a few breaths.

EXPERIENCE THE POSE
Release unconscious tension in your legs by telling your legs that they can let go and relax, especially the inner thighs and knees. Notice how the legs become heavier as you breathe naturally. Release any sense of burden you may have in your shoulders and hips as you give your body over to gravity.

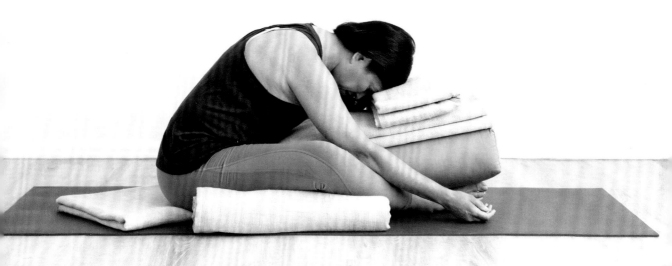

Variation

If you have difficulty bending your upper body forward to meet the support or are pregnant and require additional room for your belly, you can angle a high block underneath the bolster to create a ramp. Make sure to anchor the bolster and block securely on the mat to prevent them from slipping.

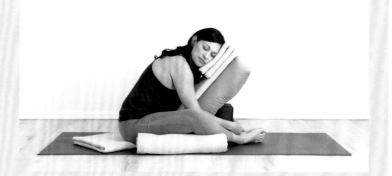

Supported Standing Wide-Legged Forward Bend

RECOMMENDED TIME // 30 SECONDS TO 1 MINUTE

As you hold yourself with ease in this standing restorative pose, you'll relieve stress and tension in the upper back and shoulders while gently opening the inner leg muscles and hamstrings.

WHAT YOU NEED
- Mat
- Blocks (2)

PRECAUTIONS
Not recommended if you have a cold or sinus infection, eye issues, a hiatal hernia, uncontrolled hypertension, or osteoporosis. Follow the Safe Practice Guidelines (p. 28) for acute sciatica or injured hamstrings. Do not practice in the last month of pregnancy.

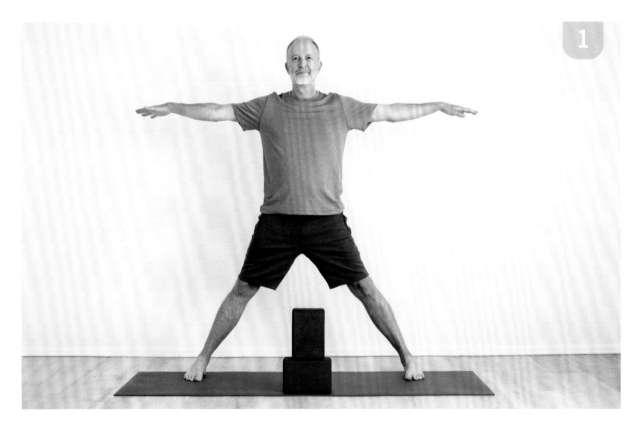

1

Stack two blocks, one medium and one high, near the front edge of the mat. Stand behind the blocks with your heels placed along the back edge of the mat. Extend your arms out to a T, taking note of the position of your wrists, then slowly step your feet outward until they're aligned underneath your wrists with your toes pointing forward. *(If needed, anchor your feet and heels against a wall to maintain balance.)*

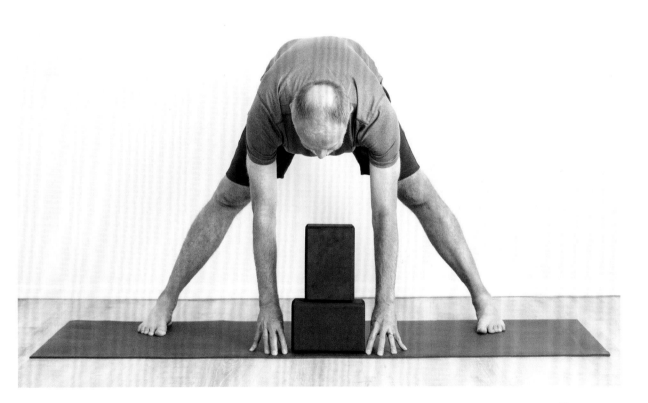

Place your hands at your hips, inhale deeply. Then exhale and drop your chin to your chest as you slowly extend your spine forward and down until your torso is nearly parallel with the floor, releasing your fingertips down to the floor and beneath your shoulders. You should sense even weight across all parts of the soles of your feet. *(If you cannot easily touch the ground with your hands, try the chair variation instead.)*

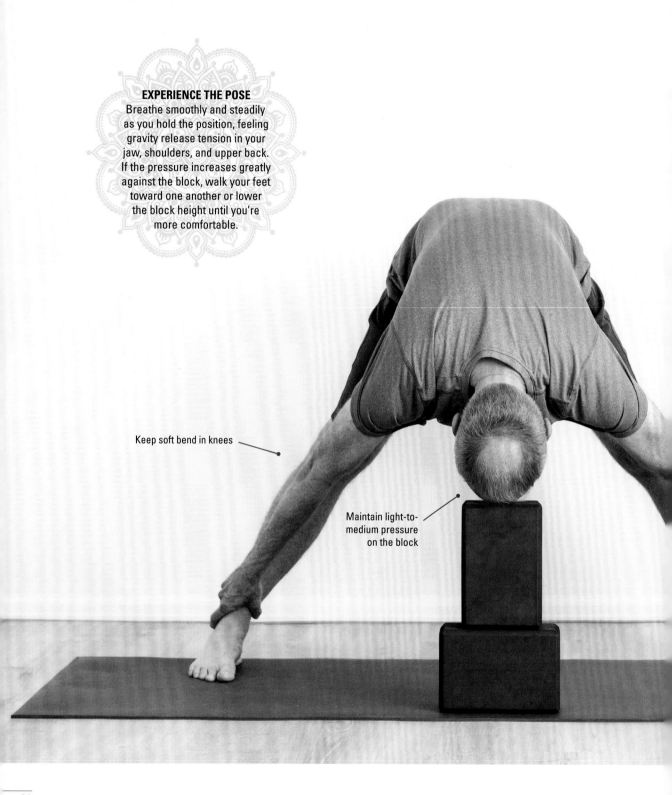

EXPERIENCE THE POSE
Breathe smoothly and steadily
as you hold the position, feeling
gravity release tension in your
jaw, shoulders, and upper back.
If the pressure increases greatly
against the block, walk your feet
toward one another or lower
the block height until you're
more comfortable.

Keep soft bend in knees

Maintain light-to-
medium pressure
on the block

3

Position the blocks under the center of your forehead then slowly lower your torso down until the block meets the scalp just above the forehead. Adjust your legs for comfort by walking your feet out or in and adjusting the block height. You should feel your tailbone descending downward to your heels while maintaining a soft lumbar spinal curve. Gently grasp your outer ankles.

TRANSITION OUT: Release your hands from your ankles and let them dangle toward the ground for a moment, then place them on your hips. Exhale and engage your abdomen and leg muscles, then inhale and slowly lift the whole spine upward without rolling your spine. Release your hands down by your sides and step the legs together. Breathe into any sensations that are present.

Variation

This variation increases stability in the legs with the aid of a chair for additional support. Secure the legs of a chair on a second mat or up against a wall. Place a square-fold blanket on the seat, then set a medium block on the blanket and toward the middle of the seat to support your forehead. Practice the pose as instructed but with your elbows and hands resting on the seat of the chair.

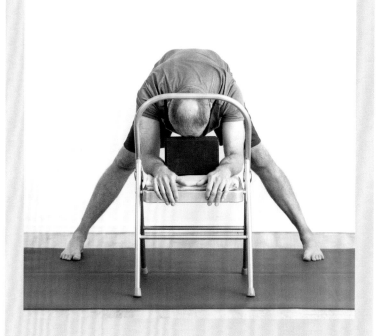

Supported Seated Angle

RECOMMENDED TIME // 3–5 MINUTES

Revive tired legs and release stale energy in the back of your body with this wide-leg forward bend. The digestive and eliminatory organs are also gently compressed and soothed here.

WHAT YOU NEED
- Mat
- Blankets (2)
  » 1 square fold
  » 1 rectangle fold
- Flat bolster
- Blocks (2)

PRECAUTIONS
Do not practice if you have a hiatal hernia. Follow the Safe Practice Guidelines (p. 28) if you have sacroiliac or knee pain. If you're pregnant or have osteoporosis, practice the variation.

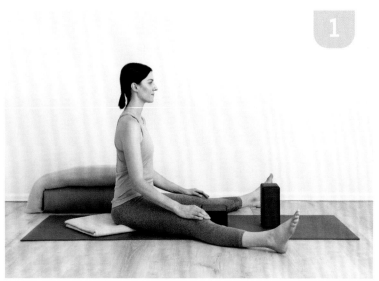

1

Place the square-fold blanket across the middle of one end of the mat, with a neatly folded corner pointing up the middle of the mat. Stack the rectangle-fold blanket on top of the bolster and place it to the side of the mat and within arm's reach. Sit on the edge of the square-fold blanket and extend your legs out in front of you, widening them into a *V* shape, but without straining your inner thighs or hips. Position a low block between your knees, and a high block between your feet. (*If your knees do not easily lower to the floor, place two square-fold or rolled blankets underneath them.*)

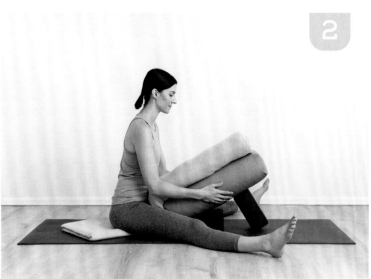

2

Create the bolster ramp by placing the bolster on the blocks with the highest end of the bolster pointed away from you. Adjust the angles of the blocks until the bolster is securely anchored to the mat. Inhale and lengthen your spine upward, then exhale and begin to slowly reach your upper body forward and down to meet the support in front of you. (*If you feel strain in your low back, or feel your low back rounding with your tailbone tucking underneath you, increase the height of the square-fold blanket.*)

3

Turn a cheek to the blanket as your upper body meets the support. Rest your arms on your legs or the ground. Your neck is elongated, and your chin is tucked slightly inward. Close your eyes, if it's comfortable.

TRANSITION OUT: Exhale and push your palms gently into the floor to lift your torso upward without rolling your spine. Press your hands into the floor behind you as you bend your knees, one at a time, and place your feet flat on the ground. Scoot backward from the bolster and collect your knees and legs, then drop your knees to one side and transition away from the props.

EXPERIENCE THE POSE
Once you arrive in the pose, stay present to ensure you are completely comfortable so your body and mind can relax. Breathe naturally. Halfway through the hold, you can switch the head to lay on the opposite cheek, if it's comfortable.

Variation

If you have difficulty bending your upper body forward to meet the support, stand a round bolster on end to provide higher support for your head. As you bend forward, place your forehead on the edge of the bolster, elongating your neck and tucking your chin slightly toward your throat. Rest your hands on your legs. Make sure to anchor the bolster securely into the mat, and add blankets under the knees if necessary.

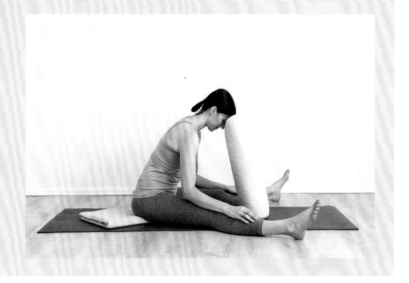

Supported Pigeon

RECOMMENDED TIME // 1–3 MINUTES

In an active yoga movement practice, Pigeon Pose is considered a challenging stretch. This restorative version, however, swaps effort for ease so you can relieve tension in your inner and outer hips while completely supporting your knees and pelvis.

WHAT YOU NEED
- Mat
- Blanket
  » long-rectangle fold
- Flat bolster
- Round bolster

PRECAUTIONS
Follow the Safe Practice Guidelines (p. 28) if you have sacroiliac pain or limited range of motion in your hips and knees. Consult a healthcare professional about a recent knee surgery or injury. Do not practice if you're more than three months pregnant.

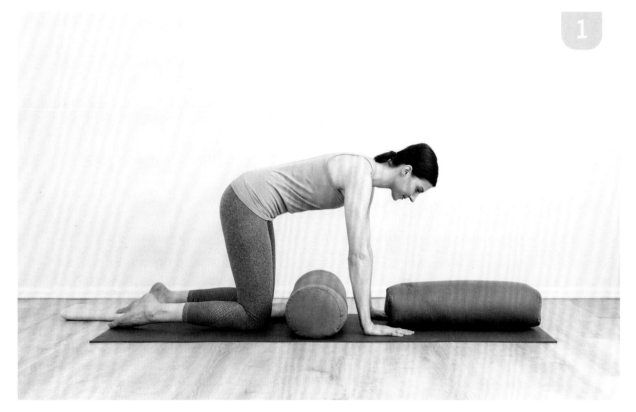

1

Position the round bolster widthwise across the middle of the mat and the flat bolster lengthwise up the center of the mat, leaving a generous hand's length of space between the bolsters. Place the long-rectangle-fold blanket on one side of the mat and just below the round bolster. Start in Table, with your left knee resting on the long-rectangle-fold blanket and your hands positioned at the base of the flat bolster.

Walk your hands forward on the mat, then step your right foot forward and over the round bolster. Walk your foot to the left as you drop your shin down into the space between the bolsters.

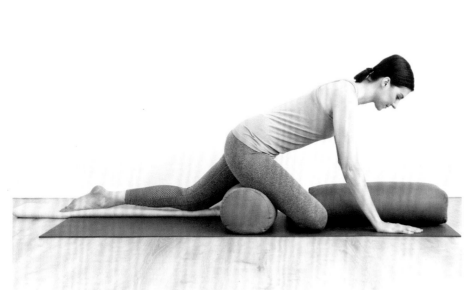

Curl your left toes under and lift your left knee off the mat, then walk your left leg back until it's fully extended. Snugly secure the round bolster underneath your pelvis, then relax your left knee and top of the left foot back to the blanket.

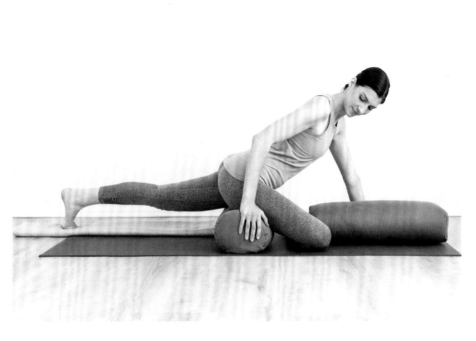

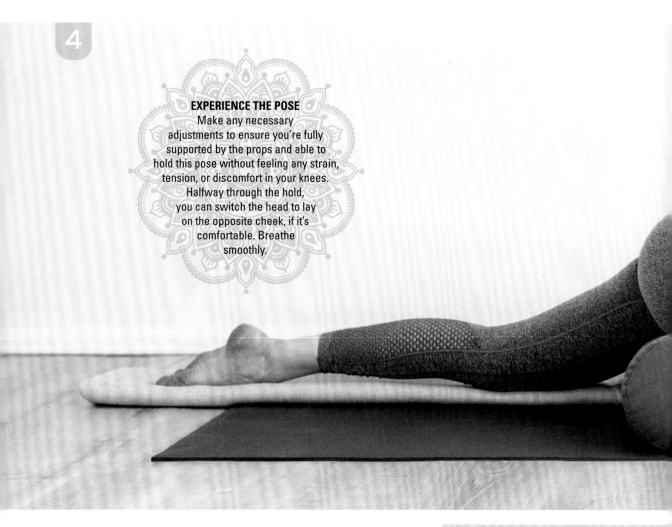

EXPERIENCE THE POSE
Make any necessary adjustments to ensure you're fully supported by the props and able to hold this pose without feeling any strain, tension, or discomfort in your knees. Halfway through the hold, you can switch the head to lay on the opposite cheek, if it's comfortable. Breathe smoothly.

Inhale and reach long through your spine from the pelvis to the crown of your head, then exhale and walk your hands forward as you lower your torso down to the support, turning one cheek to the side when you arrive at the bolster. Cradle the flat bolster with your forearms and place your palms flat on the floor in front of the bolster. *(If you experience strain in your hips when you lower your torso down, you can add two yoga blocks underneath the bolster to elevate it closer to your body. If discomfort in the hips still does not resolve, stack the round bolster on 1 or 2 rectangle-fold blankets.)*

TRANSITION OUT: Slide your hands back near your shoulders. Exhale, feel the abdomen engage lightly, and push into the palms to lift the torso. Gently lift the pelvis so you can pull the round bolster off the mat and to the left. Lift your right knee up and lengthen the right leg back alongside the left. Press to Table, but keep the right leg extended back, tucking the toes under to encourage blood flow back into the right knee, then drop your right knee to the mat. Repeat the pose on the opposite side.

Variation

If this pose isn't comfortable for your knees or hips, bend your extended leg forward to about 45 degrees until your legs resemble a pinwheel shape. Shift the end of the round bolster toward the middle of the mat and under your pelvis, making room for your back leg. Elevate the lower hip with more blankets, if necessary.

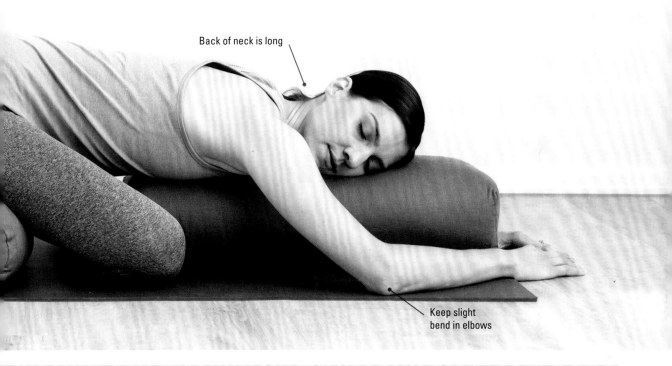

Back of neck is long

Keep slight bend in elbows

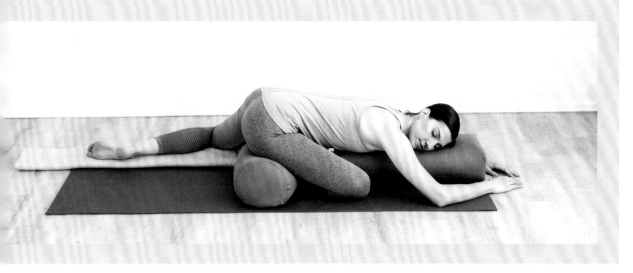

Supported Standing Forward Bend

RECOMMENDED TIME // 1–3 MINUTES

Most restorative yoga poses are practiced on the ground, but this standing pose is excellent for quieting the mind, relieving a mild headache, or opening the whole posterior chain of your body—from the soles of your feet to the crown of your head.

WHAT YOU NEED
- Mat
- Blocks (2)

PRECAUTIONS
Do not practice in the last month of pregnancy. Not recommended if you have a cold or sinus infection, eye issues, a hiatal hernia, uncontrolled hypertension, or osteoporosis. Follow the Safe Practice Guidelines (p. 28) if you have acute sciatica or injured hamstrings.

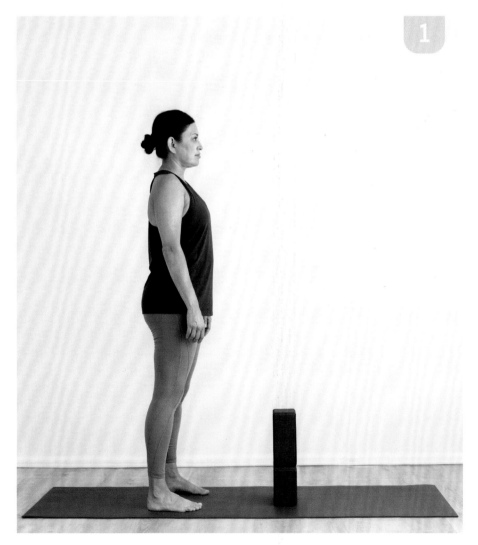

1 Stack the blocks near the middle of the mat, with a medium block placed on bottom and a high block stacked on top. Stand near the bottom end of the mat with your feet positioned wider than your hips and about shoulder-width apart, and your toes pointing forward with the outer edges of your feet parallel to the sides of the mat. *(If needed, you can anchor your buttocks and heels against a wall to maintain balance.)*

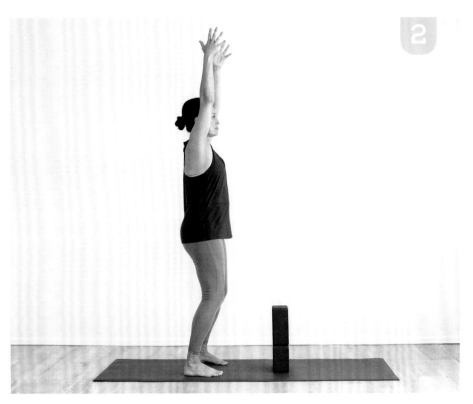

Inhale and reach your arms comfortably overhead. Create a slight bend in the knees to avoid hyperextension.

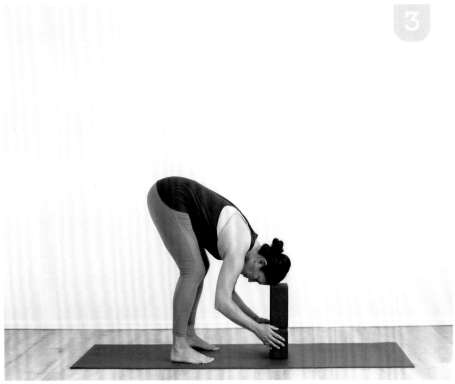

Exhale and bend forward from the hips while slowly sweeping your hands down to the floor until your head arrives at the blocks. Your head should meet the blocks at the spot on the scalp just above the forehead, where the skull begins to round. Adjust the blocks until you are comfortable and the body and mind may relax completely.

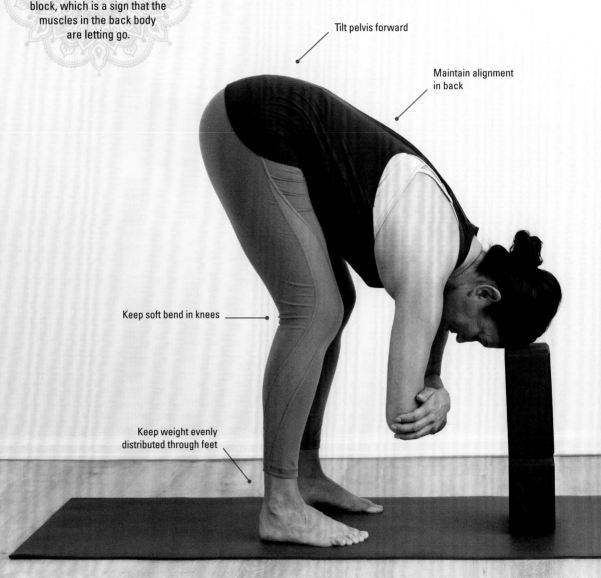

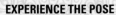

EXPERIENCE THE POSE
Release any expectations or achieving nature you may have about this pose. Breathe smoothly and stay present for the sensation of growing heaviness against the block, which is a sign that the muscles in the back body are letting go.

Tilt pelvis forward

Maintain alignment in back

Keep soft bend in knees

Keep weight evenly distributed through feet

4

Grasp the opposing elbows with your hands and let your upper body dangle toward the ground. Maintain light to medium pressure on the block, but don't rest your entire weight on the block. *(If your forehead does not easily reach the blocks, walk your feet wider, a few inches at a time, until you can comfortably rest your head on the blocks. If the pressure on your head increases greatly against the block, try walking your feet closer to one another or adjusting the block height.)*

TRANSITION OUT: Release the hold of your elbows, then place your hands on your hips. Moving slowly to avoid dizziness, come out of the pose by bending slightly into your knees, engaging your abdomen and leg muscles, and inhaling as you slowly lift your torso upward without rolling your spine. Release your hands down by your sides and stay present with the effects of the pose for a few breaths.

Variation

Try this variation if the standard pose proves to be too uncomfortable or if you experience significant rounding in the lower spine. Place a square-fold blanket on a sturdy chair, making sure the feet of the chair are secured on the mat. Practice the pose as instructed, bringing your head down to the meet the front edge of the chair. *(Add a block under the forehead to reduce strain in the legs.)*

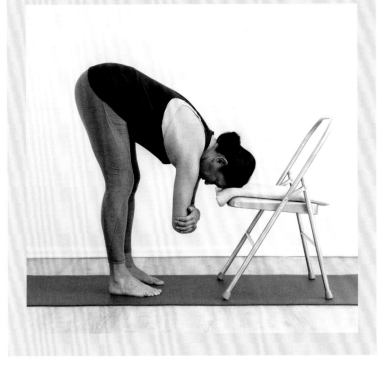

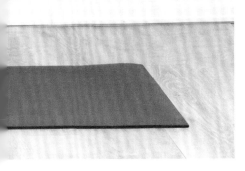

Supported Seated Forward Bend

RECOMMENDED TIME // 3-5 MINUTES

When practiced with ease, this pose focuses your attention inward to rest your mind and anchor you in the present. Surrender your upper body into the props to feel length in your back.

WHAT YOU NEED
- Mat
- Blankets (3–4)
  » 1 square fold
  » 1-2 rectangle fold
  » 1 rolled
- Flat bolster

PRECAUTIONS
Do not practice if you're pregnant or have a hiatal hernia. If you have osteoporosis, try the variation. Follow the Safe Practice Guidelines (p. 28) if you have acute sciatica or injured hamstrings.

1

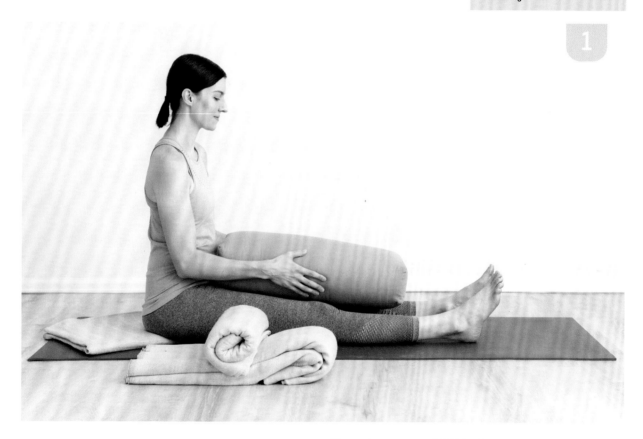

Place the square-fold blanket across the middle of one end of the mat, with a neatly folded corner pointing up the middle. Sit on the edge of the blanket with your legs extended in front of you and spaced slightly apart. Place the bolster on top of your legs. *(If your knees do not easily lower to the floor or you experience pain in your hamstrings, place a rolled blanket underneath both knees for extra support.)*

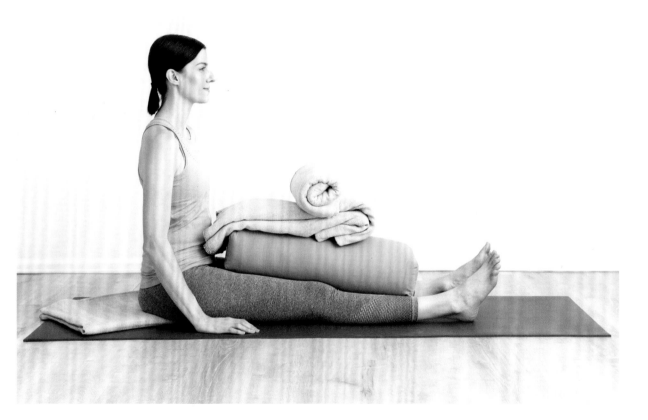

Bend forward to gauge how much space remains between you and the bolster, then begin arranging the rectangle-fold and rolled blankets on top of the bolster until you can comfortably rest your torso and head on the stack. You've arrived when you no longer feel any tension in your back or legs when bending forward.

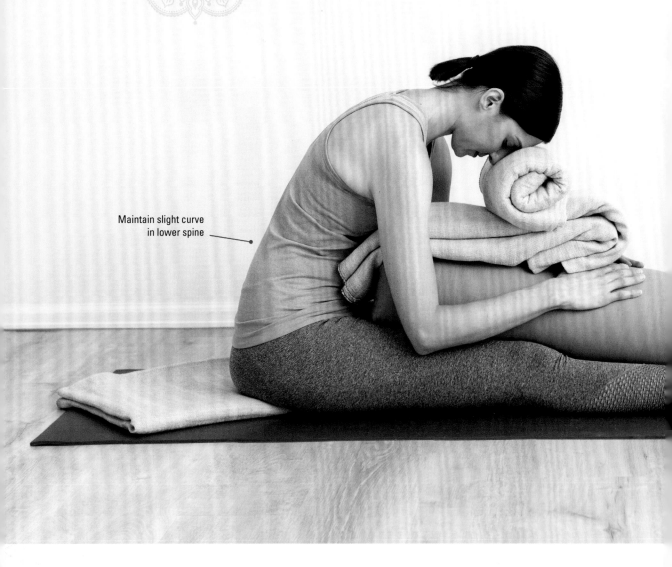

**EXPERIENCE
THE POSE**
Release tension in the
toes and all the muscles of
the legs. Breathe naturally,
feeling relaxation wash
up and down your
whole back.

Maintain slight curve
in lower spine

Inhale, lengthen your spine upward, then exhale and gently fold your upper body down to meet the support in front of you. Rest your forehead on the blanket, keeping your neck long and chin slightly tucked inward and toward the throat. Anchor your hands under the blanket and on top of the bolster so that your arms can rest without effort. Close your eyes, if it's comfortable.

TRANSITION OUT: Lower your hands to the floor. Press into your palms, then exhale and lift back into a seat. Remove the props from your legs, then bend your knees, place your palms behind you, and press down to lift the front of your chest upward. Take a few slow, deep breaths, then release.

Variation

To reduce strain in the hips and legs, try this variation that requires only one leg be extended at a time. Place one foot against the opposite inner thigh, and position the extended leg outward at a slight angle from the hip. *(If the knee hovers above the ground, wedge a square-fold blanket underneath.)* Arrange the props inside the extended leg. Hold for 3 to 5 minutes on one side before switching to the opposite side.

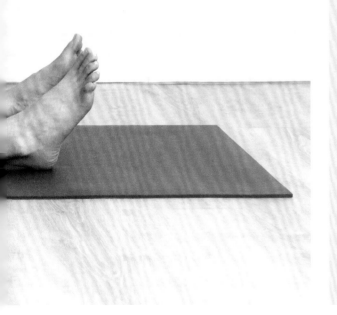

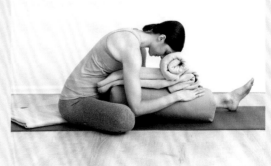

Supported Seated Forward Bend
with chair

RECOMMENDED TIME // 2–3 MINUTES

There are two ways to approach this calming forward bend, and both will soothe stiff shoulders, while relaxing the neck and elongating the spine. This position gifts you a few minutes of rest and doesn't require many props, making it easy to practice on-the-go or even at a desk.

WHAT YOU NEED
- Mat
- Chair
- Blanket
  - » 1 square fold

PRECAUTIONS
Not recommended if you have a cold or sinus infection, eye issues, a hiatal hernia, indigestion, or uncontrolled hypertension. If you're pregnant, practice the variation.

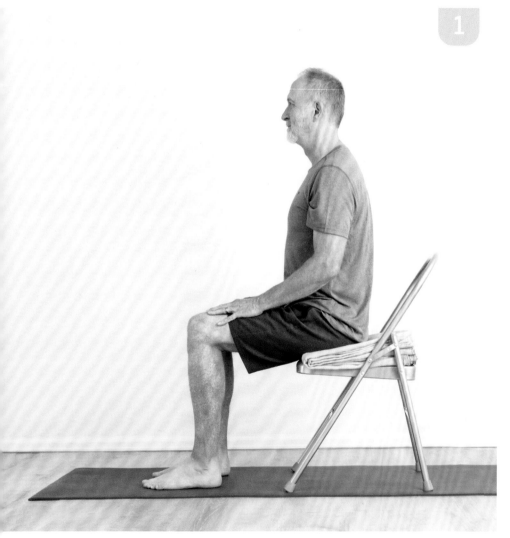

1

Sit on your buttocks at the edge of the chair. Step your feet directly under your knees, with your toes pointing forward, and about 8 inches (20cm) of space between the feet. Rest your hands on your thighs.

EXPERIENCE THE POSE

As you turn your senses inward, become aware of the effects of gravity on your bones. When breathing in, feel the breath spread horizontally across your back; when breathing out, allow your head and arms to hang freely.

Deeply inhale and lift up through your spine and the crown of your head, then exhale and slowly lower your upper body down to your thighs as you release your arms and head down to the floor. Stack your hands with palms facing up. Close your eyes, if it's comfortable.

TRANSITION OUT:
First move your hands to the outer edges of the chair seat, then exhale and slowly lift your torso upright without rolling your spine. Spend a few moments breathing easily with your head above the heart.

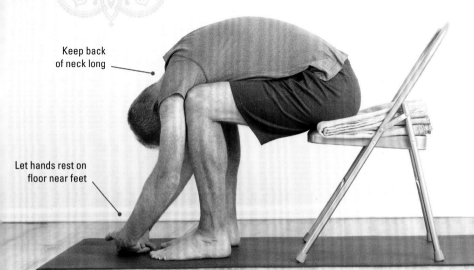

Keep back of neck long

Let hands rest on floor near feet

Variation

Reduce back and neck strain with this variation. Place a square-fold blanket on the mat and a second square-fold blanket on the chair. Sit cross-legged on the blanket, lean forward, and stack your hands on top of one another on the chair, then lower your forehead down to the seat. Stay for 2–3 minutes, then change the cross of your legs and repeat.

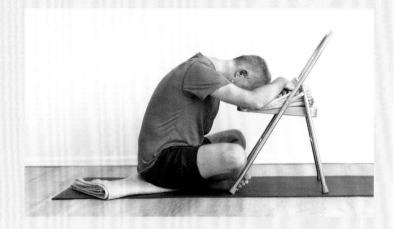

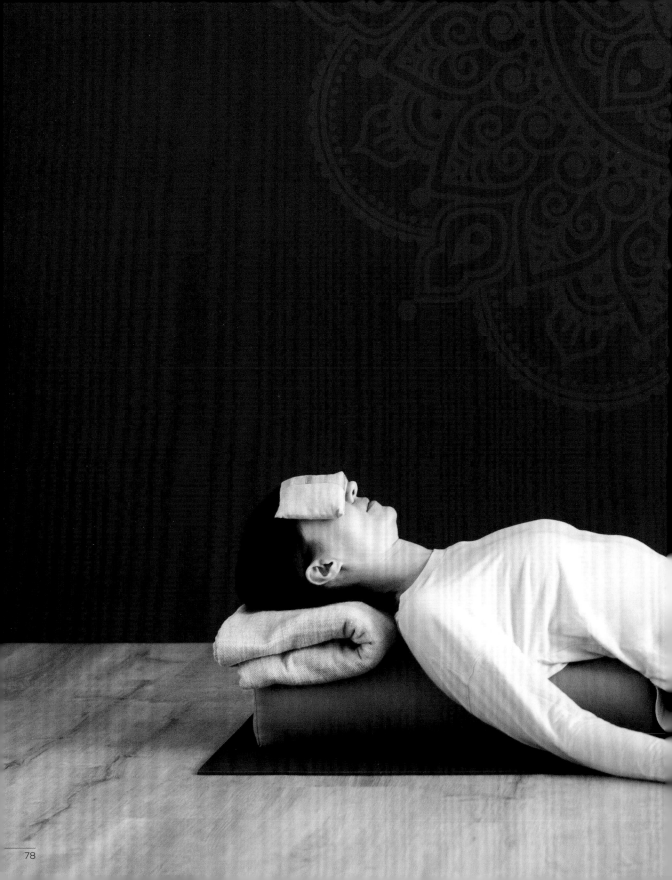

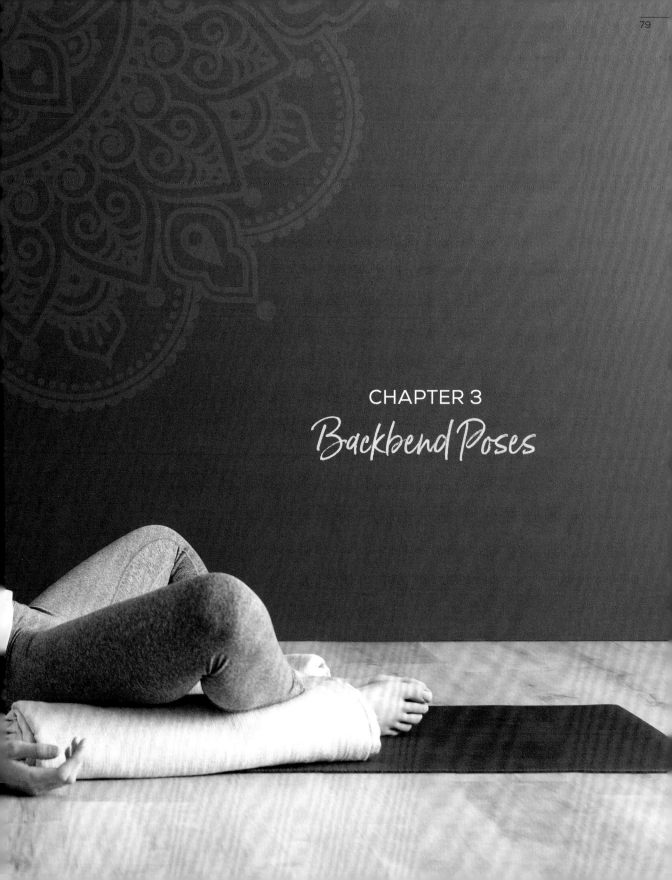

CHAPTER 3

Backbend Poses

Constructive Rest Position

RECOMMENDED TIME // 10-20 MINUTES

This pose releases and relaxes the psoas, the muscle that connects the upper and lower body from the spine to the legs. If tight, the psoas can contribute to back pain and also make deep breathing difficult. Practiced regularly, this position can decompress the spine, relieve back pain, and minimize the effects of emotional and physical stress.

WHAT YOU NEED
- Mat
- Blanket
- Block
- Hand towel
- Looped strap

PRECAUTIONS
Do not practice if you are more than three months pregnant.

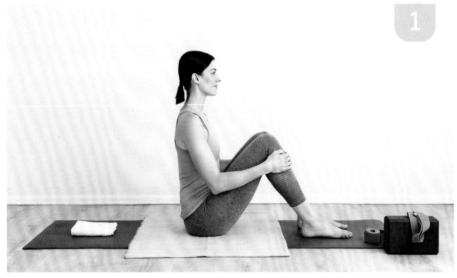

1

Fold the blanket in half twice and place it across the center of the mat. Fold the hand towel widthwise three times to make a small square, then position it at the top edge of the mat. Place the block and looped strap off to one side. Sit on the blanket with your knees bent and positioned hip-distance apart. Place your feet flat on the mat with your toes pointing forward.

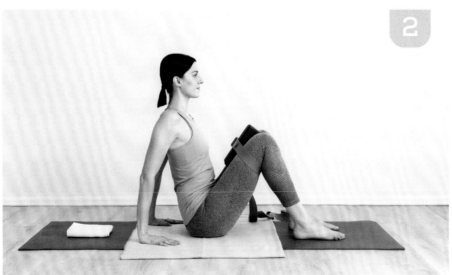

2

Slip the looped strap over your feet and up over your knees. Place the block between your inner thighs with the widest sides against your legs, then tighten the strap around your outer thighs. Place your hands on the floor and begin lowering down onto your back by lengthening your spine, while avoiding rounding your spine as you recline.

EXPERIENCE THE POSE
Breathe naturally and tell your body to relax its grip at the hips. You may feel like the pelvis or legs are "moving" as your muscles relax and rebalance. Allow any tension in your body to release in its own time. There is nothing that you need to do to make this happen, just allow yourself to be.

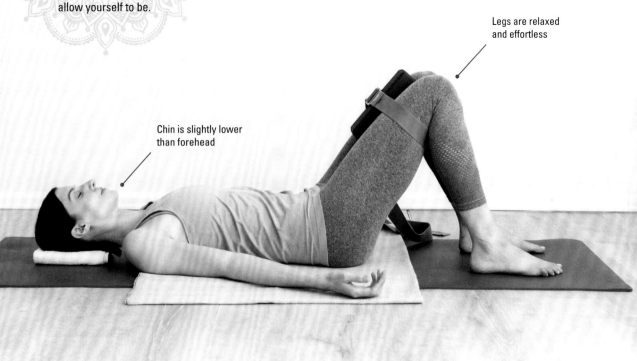

Legs are relaxed and effortless

Chin is slightly lower than forehead

Position the hand towel under the base of your skull, but not underneath your neck, and adjust the height for comfort. Walk your feet forward until you feel an equal balance of pressure throughout the soles of your feet. Your thighs should be parallel so that the knees are neither falling inward or outward, and your legs and abdomen should be completely relaxed without any effort or holding. Rest your arms by your sides with your palms facing up.

TRANSITION OUT: Remove the props from your legs, then slowly extend your legs until they're flat on the floor. Observe how the back and legs feel against the floor. Roll to one side and rest for a few breaths before sitting up.

Simple Supported Backbend

RECOMMENDED TIME // 1-4 MINUTES

Ease arrives through simplicity. You can reclaim openness in your breath, calm your busy mind, and relieve tension in your upper back and shoulders simply by lying on your back and doing nothing. Practice this restorative backbend to counteract your everyday experiences of sitting or rushing from one task to another.

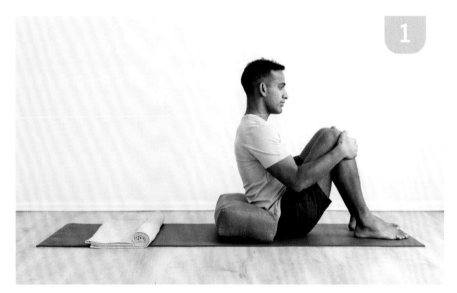

1 Place the bolster widthwise across the middle of the mat, and place the half-rolled blanket at the top of the mat and about 8–10 inches (20–25cm) away from the bolster, with the rolled portion closest to the bolster. Sit on the mat with your low back against the bolster, your knees bent and upright, and your feet flat on the ground.

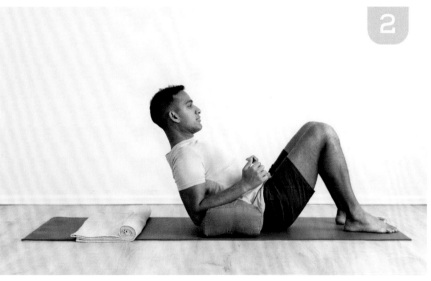

2 Recline and hook your elbows to the back edge of the bolster. Inhale and press forward into the bolster to elongate the front of your torso, feeling your spine lengthen up and back.

EXPERIENCE THE POSE
With your arms wide and
whole body relaxed, receive
the spacious feeling that may
arise in the chest. Feel
completely held and give all
effort over to the ground.

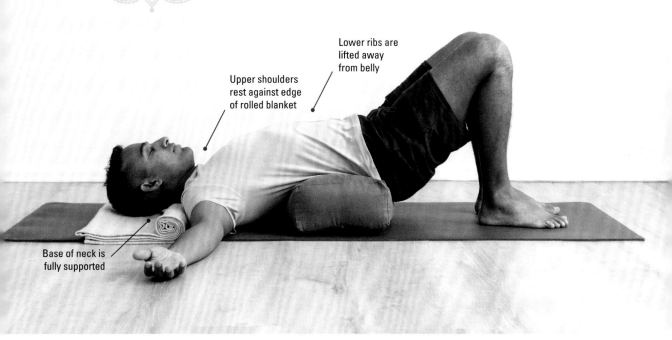

Lower ribs are
lifted away
from belly

Upper shoulders
rest against edge
of rolled blanket

Base of neck is
fully supported

Exhale and lower your upper body backward and down, resting your head just beyond the roll of the blanket with the rolled portion touching your shoulders. Let your buttocks hang slightly off the bolster's edge. Widen your feet and rest with your knees open or gently touching, and walk your feet forward or backward to find the spot that feels best. Reach your arms out to a *T*, with palms facing up. Apply the eye pillow or close your eyes, if it's comfortable. *(If your neck feels crushed against the floor, increase the height of the bolster by stacking another blanket on top. You may also choose to increase or decrease the blanket roll under your neck.)*

TRANSITION OUT: Lift your head slightly and slide the blanket roll off the mat. Exhale and gently push into the feet to slide your upper body backward and off the bolster. Reach your hands down and slowly push the bolster until it's underneath your knees. Stay for three easy breaths, observing any sensations, then roll to one side and sit up.

Mountain Brook

RECOMMENDED TIME // 5-15 MINUTES

This backbend offers rejuvenation and relief for tight muscles caused by a tendency to slouch during everyday activities. By gently opening the upper chest as well as the abdominal muscles and diaphragm, you'll expand your capacity to breathe deeper throughout your lungs. Practice to embody calm energy, improve posture, elevate a low mood, and relieve tension in the heart and throat.

WHAT YOU NEED
- Mat
- Blankets (3)
  » 1 basic fold
  » 2 rectangle fold
- Round bolster

PRECAUTIONS
Follow the Safe Practice Guidelines (p. 28) if you experience back or neck pain. Do not practice if you are more than three months pregnant.

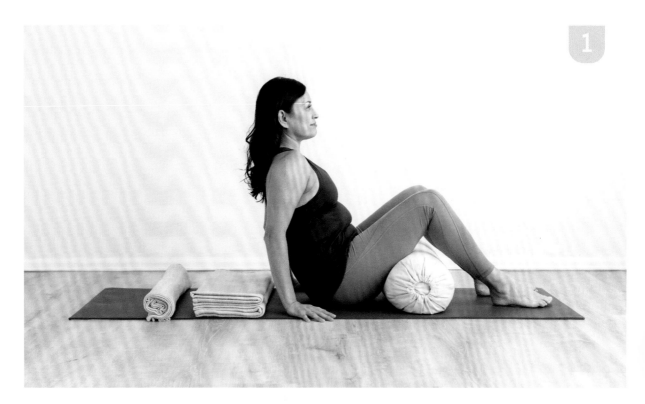

1

Roll up the basic-fold blanket from the longest side. Stack the rectangle-fold blankets near the top third of the mat, then place the rolled blanket about 4 inches (10cm) above the stack. Position the round bolster widthwise across the opposite end of the mat. Sit between the bolster and the blankets with your knees draped over the bolster and your hands flat on the mat. Begin reclining, while avoiding rounding your spine.

EXPERIENCE THE POSE
Relax your forehead, cheeks, jaw, tongue, and lips. With a few slow exhalations, allow a feeling of effortlessness to spread through your throat, upper chest, navel, and pit of the abdomen. Arrive like a pebble resting undisturbed at the bottom of a freshwater mountain brook. Breathe naturally.

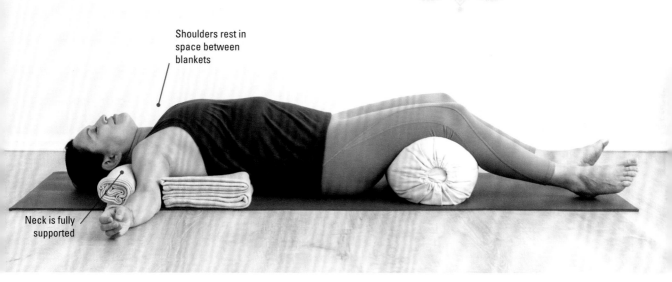

Shoulders rest in space between blankets

Neck is fully supported

Once you arrive at the blankets, slide your back up or down until you find the "just right" position. Apply the eye pillow or close your eyes, if it's comfortable. Extend your arms outward to a *T* shape, with your pinky fingers resting on the floor or your palms facing up. *(If resting with your chin tipped higher than your forehead is uncomfortable, adjust the rolled blanket so that your chin is level with your forehead. If you experience back pain, remove one rectangle blanket and place it on top of the bolster and under your knees.)*

TRANSITION OUT: Exhale and bend your knees to place your feet on the bolster. Push the bolster away and drop your knees to one side. Let your body roll heavily to the same side and use your hands to gently push your upper body up to sitting.

Supported Reclining Bound Angle

RECOMMENDED TIME // 10–15 MINUTES

Known as one of the most important poses in the restorative practice, this highly relaxing position reduces stress while gently opening the pelvis, abdomen, and chest. During and after practice you may experience a surge of well-being and peace.

WHAT YOU NEED
- Mat
- Blankets (6)
  » 3 rectangle fold
  » 1 square fold
  » 2 rolled
- Flat bolster
- Eye pillow (optional)

PRECAUTIONS
Follow the Safe Practice Guidelines (p. 28) if you experience back pain or acute sacroiliac pain. If you are more than three months pregnant, practice the version with a ramped bolster.

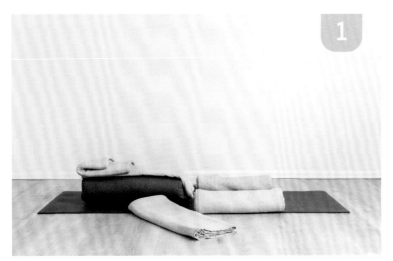

1 Position the bolster lengthwise near the top of the mat and then place a rectangle-fold blanket on top of the bolster. Place the square-fold blanket, folded down by one-third, on the top end of the bolster. Position one rectangle-fold blanket on each side of the mat and angled 45-degrees outward from the middle of the bolster, then place two rolled blankets lengthwise along the edges of the mat and near the bolster.

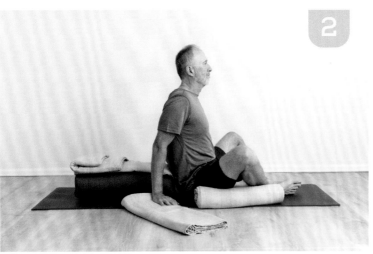

2 Sit on the mat with your low back pressed directly against the end of the bolster. Bend your knees, gently drop your thighs outward, and bring the soles of the feet together so that your feet are no closer than 12 inches (30cm) from your pelvis. Pull the two rolled blankets in to fully support your thighs and calves. Use your hands to support your body as you carefully begin to lower your upper body down to the bolster. *(If the inner thighs feel like they're stretching, add additional blankets under the legs to build up the support until the legs feel effortless.)*

Once you arrive at the bolster, adjust the square-fold blanket so that your head and neck feel fully supported. Apply the eye pillow or close your eyes, if it's comfortable. Extend your arms out on top of the blankets with your palms facing up. *(If you experience low back discomfort, pull the blanket on top of the bolster down to the space directly beneath your tailbone.)*

TRANSITION OUT: Moving as if through honey, fully extend your legs, one at a time. Exhale and then exert just enough effort to press into your palms and push your torso up to a seated position, keeping your chin tucked toward your chest for support.

EXPERIENCE THE POSE
A profound feeling of wholeness may arrive in this position if you stay present to the act of doing less and allow the whole body to release down into its support. Let the jaw hang toward the heart, and wipe all tension from your face as you breathe smoothly.

Chin is slightly higher than sternum

Sternum is slightly higher than pelvis

Variation

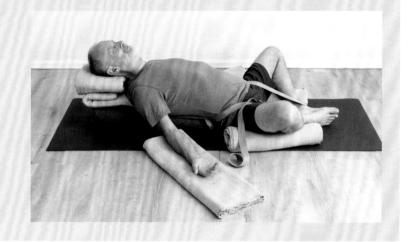

This variation will provide more support for your feet and create a sensation of being cradled. Set up the position as before, but drop a looped strap down over your torso and just below your waist, then reach the strap underneath your feet to hold the outer ankles. As you lean back, adjust the strap until the feet feel comfortably held.

Supported Reclining Bound Angle with ramped bolster

RECOMMENDED TIME // 10-15 MINUTES

Offering its own flavor of deep relaxation, this variation of an essential restorative yoga pose may be helpful if you tend to cough or fall asleep while lying down. Practice this pose as a portal to increased feelings of spaciousness and calm.

WHAT YOU NEED
- Mat
- Blankets (6)
  » 1 square fold
  » 1 rectangle fold
  » 4 rolled
- Blocks (2)
- Flat bolster
- Eye pillow (optional)

PRECAUTIONS
Follow the Safe Practice Guidelines (p. 28) if you experience knee pain or acute sacroiliac pain.

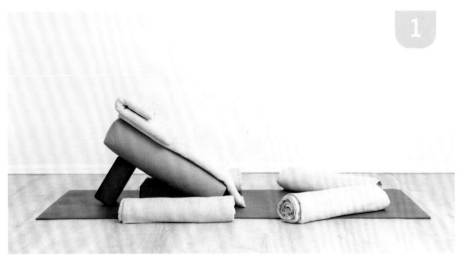

1 Position one high block and one low block near the top of the mat, then ramp the bolster up the blocks with the top block angled against the bolster. Place the rectangle-fold blanket on top of the bolster, then fold the square-fold blanket down by two-thirds and place it at the top of the ramp. Place two rolled blankets alongside the ramp, and two near the bottom of the mat.

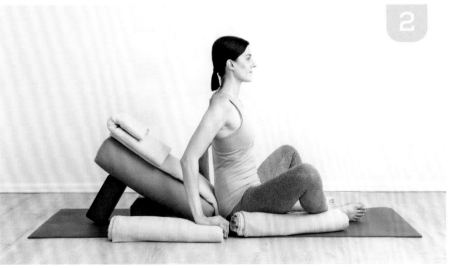

2 Sit in the center of the mat with your low back resting against the end of the ramp. Bend your knees, gently drop your thighs outward, and bring the soles of your feet together so that your feet are no closer than 12 inches (30cm) from your pelvis. Pull the rolled blankets at the bottom of the mat in to fully support your thighs and calves. Use your hands for support as you lower down onto the bolster.

3

EXPERIENCE THE POSE
Rest in the *not doing* after
all the doing of setting up this
position. Just simply let your
body breathe and be, and stay
present to any sensations
that arrive.

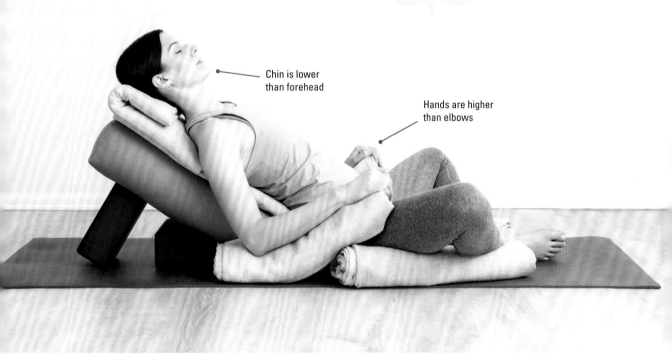

Chin is lower
than forehead

Hands are higher
than elbows

Once you arrive at the bolster, adjust the square-fold blanket so that your
head and neck are fully supported and your forehead is higher than your chin.
Lift one end of each rolled armrest blanket onto the tops of the blankets placed
under your legs. Apply the eye pillow or close your eyes, if it's comfortable. Place
your forearms on top of the rolled blankets with your palms facing down and
your fingers resting over the lips of the blankets. *(If you desire more warmth
and comfort, place an additional basic-fold blanket over the top of the lower
abdomen and legs. If you experience low back discomfort, pull the blanket on
top of the bolster down to the space directly beneath your tailbone.)*

TRANSITION OUT: Slowly straighten your legs, one at a time. Exhale, place your
palms on the floor, then push your upper body up into a seated position. Take your
time to acquaint yourself with the space around you before moving on.

Supported Reclining Pose

RECOMMENDED TIME // 10–15 MINUTES

If your knees and hips are uncomfortable when you practice Supported Reclining Bound Angle, you can try this variation. Like its predecessors, this position is supremely stress relieving and also supports women's bodies during menstruation, pregnancy, and menopause.

WHAT YOU NEED
- Mat
- Blankets (5)
  » 1 square fold
  » 1 rectangle fold
  » 3 rolled
- Blocks (2)
- Flat bolster
- Round bolster
- Eye pillow (optional)

PRECAUTIONS
This feels best if your lower back is fully supported.

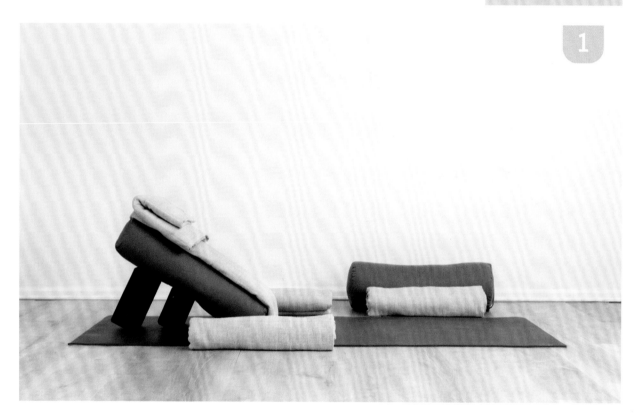

1

Place two yoga blocks, one high and one medium, at the top end of the mat, then ramp the bolster lengthwise up the blocks, angling the blocks against the bolster at 45-degree angles as you do so. Place the rectangle-fold blanket on top of the bolster, then fold the square-fold blanket down by two-thirds and place it at the top of the bolster. Position one rolled blanket on each side of the mat and next to the bolster. Place the third rolled blanket and round bolster next to the bottom end of the mat.

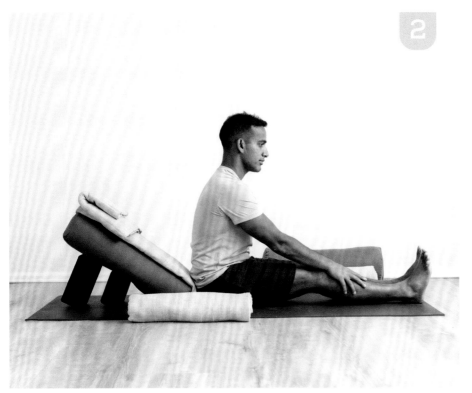

2 Sit on the mat with your legs extended in front of you. Lean forward, then scoot backward until your hips are positioned directly against the base of the ramp.

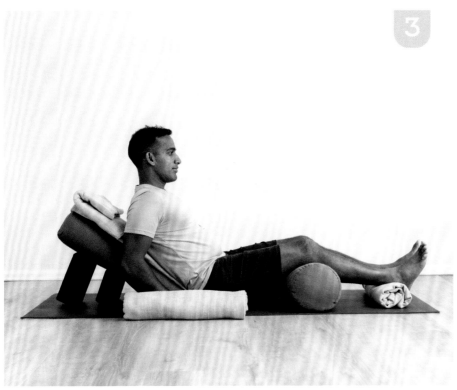

3 Place the round bolster under your knees and the rolled blanket under your ankles with your heels hanging over the edge of the blanket. Use your hands for support as you begin to lower your upper body down onto the ramp.

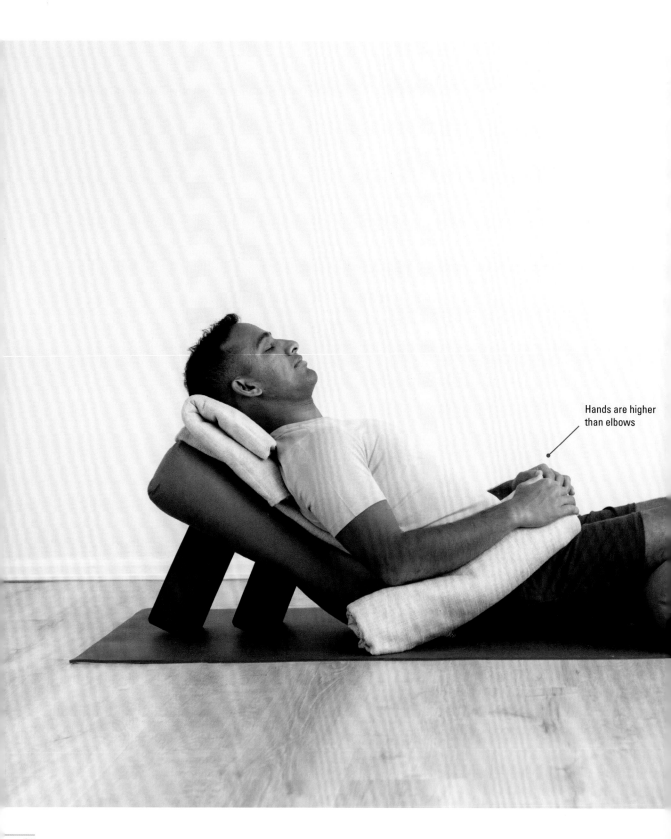

Hands are higher
than elbows

4

EXPERIENCE THE POSE

Surrender your attention to the deep stillness arriving in the body with every breath. Allow the breath to move as it wants naturally, giving your thoughts permission to come and go. Become the one who is watching this process without judgment or reaction.

Once you arrive at the bolster, adjust the blanket so that your head and neck are fully supported and your forehead is higher than your chin. Lift one end of each rolled armrest blanket onto the tops of the thighs. Apply the eye pillow or close your eyes, if it's comfortable. Place your forearms on top of the rolled blankets with your palms facing down and your fingers resting over the lips of the blankets. *(If you experience low back discomfort, pull the blanket on top of the bolster down to the space directly beneath your tailbone.)*

TRANSITION OUT: Slowly move your palms down to the floor, then exhale and push your torso upright. Bend your knees one at a time, placing your feet on the floor. Pull the bolster out from underneath your legs. If it's comfortable, sit cross-legged for a few breaths and bask in the lingering sensations of deep relaxation.

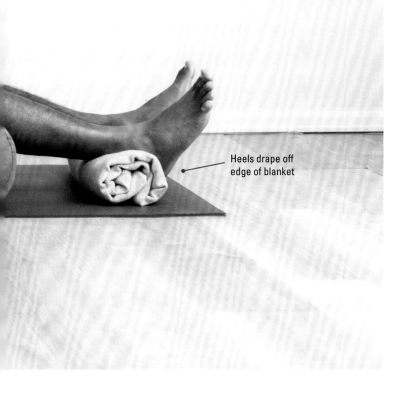

Heels drape off edge of blanket

Supported Fish

RECOMMENDED TIME // 3-5 MINUTES

This pose offers a gateway to feelings of lightness and releases a sense of burden and responsibility from the heart and shoulders. It can be practiced with different prop combinations depending on the level of support you desire in your back.

WHAT YOU NEED
- Mat
- Blanket
  » 1 double-square fold
- Flat bolster
- Eye pillow (optional)

PRECAUTIONS
Follow the Safe Practice Guidelines (p. 28) if you experience back pain. Do not practice if more than three months pregnant.

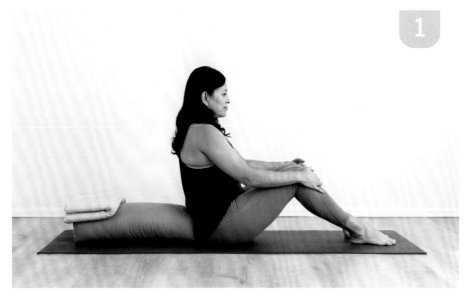

1 Position the bolster lengthwise at the top end of the mat and stack the double-square–fold blanket on the top end of the bolster. Sit on the mat with your back directly against the end of the bolster, with your knees bent and feet flat on the mat.

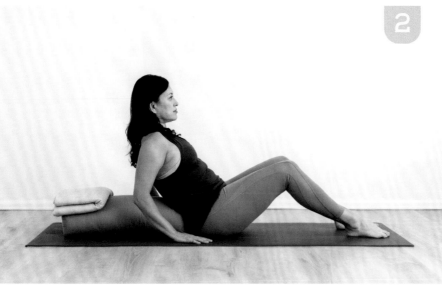

2 Place your hands on the mat for support. Inhale and lift your spine upward, then exhale and begin reclining back to the bolster.

Once you reach the bolster, adjust the blanket to ensure your head is fully supported. Apply the eye pillow or close your eyes, if it's comfortable. Extend your legs to the floor, then rest your forearms on the floor by the bolster with your palms facing up.

TRANSITION OUT: Bend your knees and plant your feet flat into the floor. Carefully roll to one side and off the props, or exhale and use your hands to slowly push up to sitting.

EXPERIENCE THE POSE
Breathe quietly, become still in the pose, and relax all effort.

Chin is lower than forehead

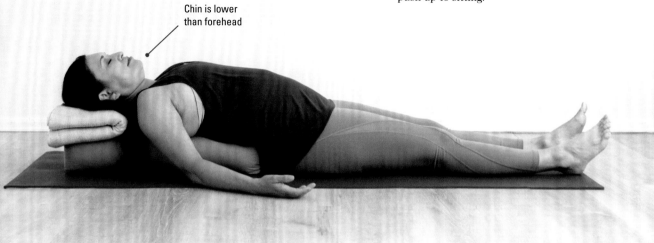

Variation

If you encounter lower back pain with this pose, try this variation instead. Practice as before, but position a round bolster across the mat and underneath your knees. If your back pain is still present in the final pose, use blankets to add more height to the bolster underneath your knees. Once you feel comfortable, add a rolled blanket underneath the backs of your ankles.

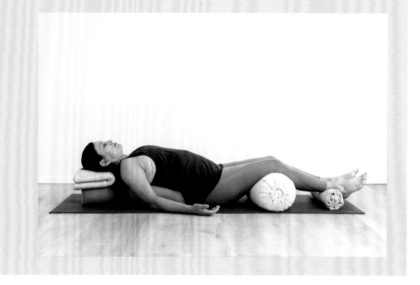

Supported Reclining Hero

RECOMMENDED TIME // 3-5 MINUTES

Embrace the feeling of lightness and expansion in the chest, lungs, hips, and legs that comes with this supported backbend. The pose counteracts the effects of sitting and may reduce back pain, enhance breathing, improve digestion, and lessen symptoms of anxiety.

WHAT YOU NEED
- Mat
- Blankets (4)
  » 1 double-square fold
  » 3 rectangle fold
- Flat bolster
- Eye pillow (optional)

PRECAUTIONS
Follow the Safe Practice Guidelines (p. 28) if you have limited range of motion in knees and ankles. Consult a healthcare professional if you've had a recent knee surgery or injury. Do not practice if you're more than three months pregnant.

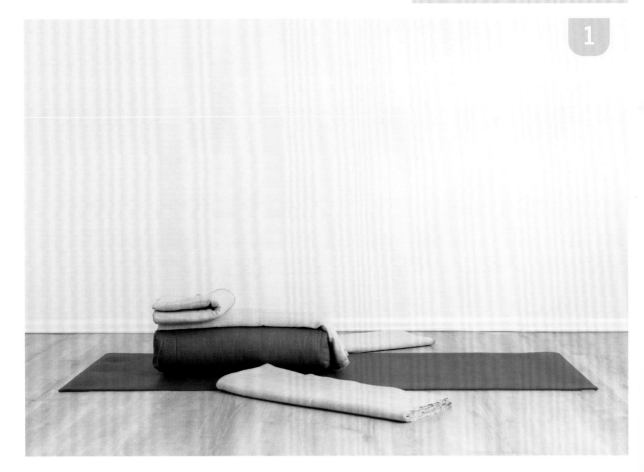

1

Position the flat bolster lengthwise near the top of the mat. Place the rectangle-fold blanket on top of the bolster, adjusting it to hang off the edge of the bolster and touch the floor. Set the double-square-fold blanket at the top end of the bolster, then place the rectangle-fold blankets at each side of the bolster, angled diagonally to support the arms.

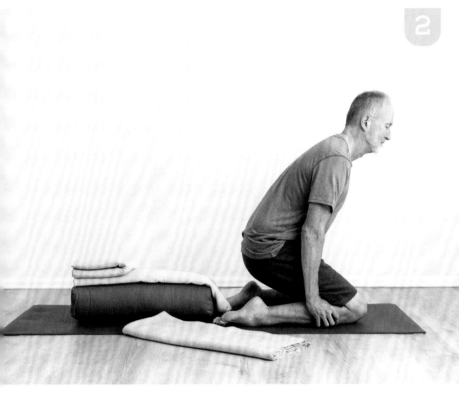

2

Kneel on the mat with the tops of your feet flat on the mat and your back to the bolster. Place your hands on your calf muscles and gently pull the muscles backward and slightly outward as you lower your hips down to the floor. Release your hands by your sides. *(If your knees are uncomfortable, roll up the end of the rectangle-fold blanket and sit on it just in front of the bolster. If your feet are uncomfortable, come out of the position and place a half-rolled blanket across the mat and underneath your ankles to elevate the ankles and toes.)*

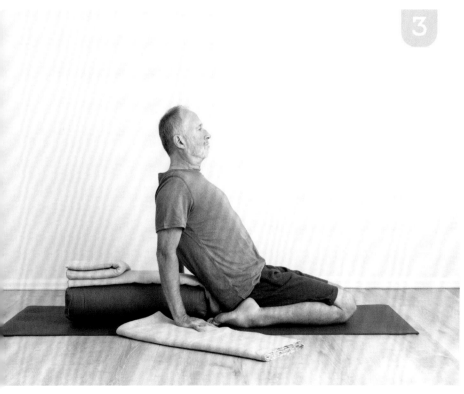

3

Adjust your knees slightly apart to resolve any back tension but not farther than outer hip distance apart. Press your hands into the floor, inhale, then lift your hips slightly off the ground as you tilt your pelvis forward. Your buttocks and tailbone should lengthen toward your knees, and your lower abdomen and navel should drop inward toward your spine until your upper body is at a 45-degree angle to the floor. Exhale and use your hands and forearms for support as you begin to lower your upper body down onto the bolster.

4

Once you reach the bolster, adjust the double-square-fold blanket to ensure your head is fully supported. Apply the eye pillow or close your eyes, if it's comfortable. Place your forearms on the rectangle-fold blankets, with your elbows and wrists supported and your palms facing up.

TRANSITION OUT: Exhale deeply and feel the depth of the exhale engage your abdominal muscles so that you may sit up safely. Keeping your chin slightly tucked, push into your hands and lift your torso back to sitting. Raise your hips and come into Table with your palms underneath your shoulders. Stretch one leg back at a time, tucking the toes under on the floor to encourage circulation throughout the legs and the knee joints. When you feel like your legs are awake, transition to a seat or a standing position.

EXPERIENCE THE POSE
Give yourself full permission to stay present with each breath as your thighs and hips settle toward the floor. Feel your breath expanding your ribcage on the inhalations, creating a sense of buoyancy in the chest on the exhalations. (Because this can be an intense opening for the front of your body, you are free to come out of the posture at any time.)

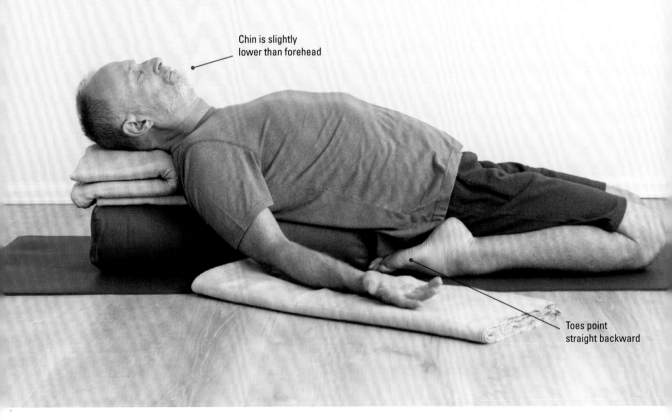

Chin is slightly lower than forehead

Toes point straight backward

Variation with ramped bolster

If the standard pose causes discomfort in the back or legs, try this variation instead. Place one tall block at the top of the mat and a short block about 6 inches (15cm) from the tall block and closer to the middle of the mat. Ramp the bolster on the blocks and add double-rectangle-fold blankets for armrests. Practice the pose as instructed.

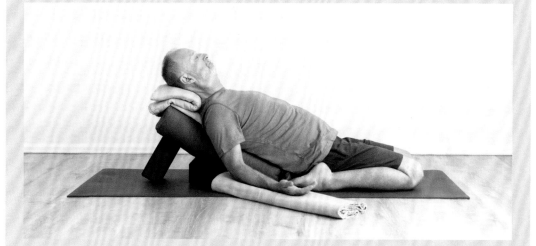

Variation: Half Hero

If bending both knees is too intense of an opening, try practicing with only one knee bent. Sit with your back to the bolster and both legs extended, then lean to the left hip, bend the right knee, and sweep the leg back toward your buttocks. Place a basic- or square-fold blanket under the left hip to make it level with the right hip.

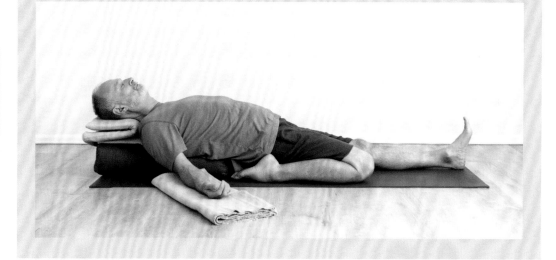

Supported Reclining Hero
with chair

RECOMMENDED TIME // 3-5 MINUTES

This variation honors your physical body by adding height to your torso so you can truly discover relaxation. Set aside any mental judgments about your body's capabilities, and know that meeting yourself where you're at is the ultimate act of self-care.

WHAT YOU NEED
- Mat
- Blankets (4)
  » 2 square fold
  » 2 rolled
- Blocks (2)
- Flat bolster
- Round bolster
- Chair

PRECAUTIONS
Follow the Safe Practice Guidelines (p. 28) if you have limited range of motion in your knees and ankles. Consult a healthcare professional if you've had a recent knee surgery or injury.

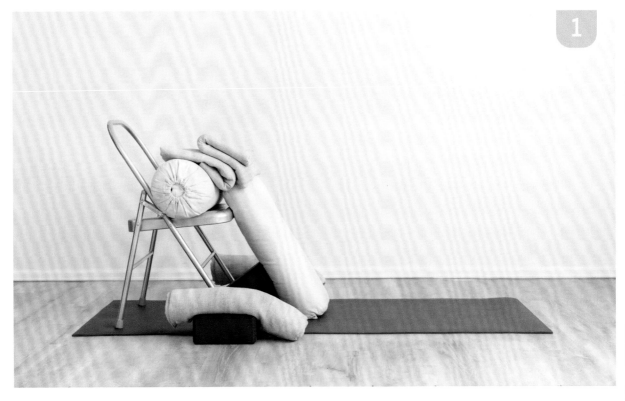

1

Position the chair so all four feet are securely on the mat. Ramp the flat bolster up the chair at a 60-degree angle, with a high-angled block wedged behind the bolster to prevent it from sagging. Place the round bolster widthwise across the chair, then place two square-fold blankets over the top of the round and flat bolsters to create a nest for your head. Position two low blocks on each side of the flat bolster, then place a rolled blanket on top of each block.

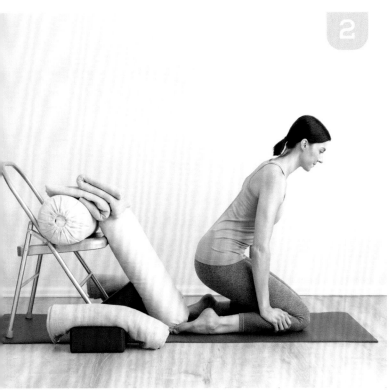

2 Kneel on the mat with your back to the bolster and the tops of the feet flat on the mat. Place your hands on your calf muscles, then gently pull backward and slightly outward to create space at the knee joints as you lower your hips down to rest in the space between your feet.

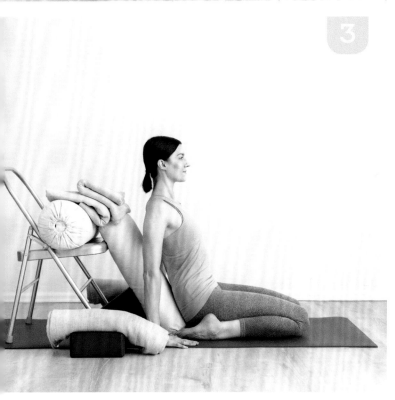

3 Release your hands and rest them along your sides. Adjust your knees slightly apart to resolve back tension, but not farther than outer hip distance apart. Press your hands into the floor, inhale, then lift the hips slightly off the ground, tilting your pelvis so that your buttocks and tailbone lengthen toward your knees, and your lower abdomen and navel drop inward toward your spine.
(If the knees are still uncomfortable, sit on a square blanket. If the feet are uncomfortable, come out of the position and place a half-rolled blanket across the mat and underneath your ankles to elevate the ankles and toes above the floor.)

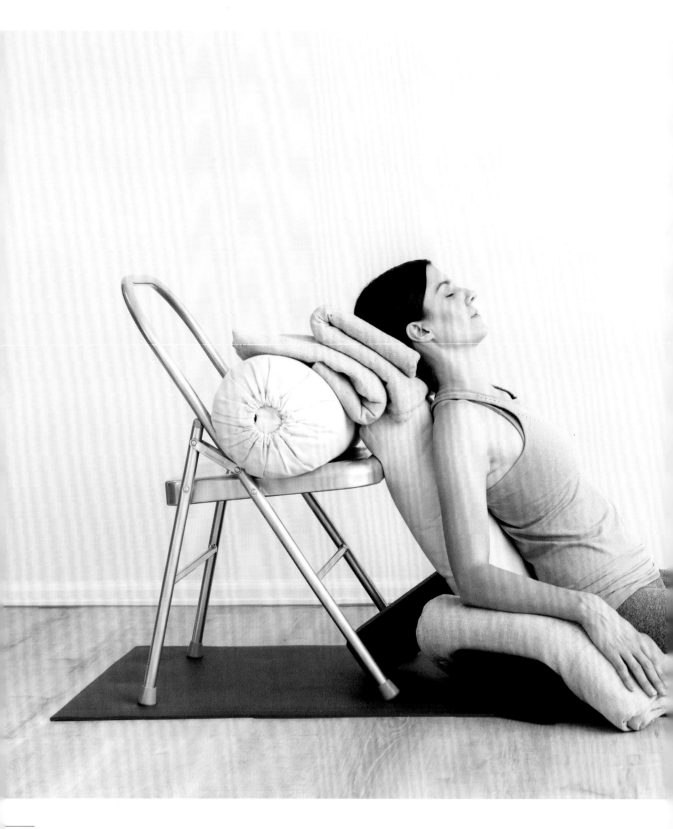

4 Exhale and lower your back to the bolster and head to the blanket. Pull the blocks and blankets in toward your body at 45-degree angles. Place your elbows, forearms, and wrists on top of the blocks and blankets. Close your eyes, if it's comfortable.

TRANSITION OUT: Exhale deeply and feel the abdominal muscles engage, then use your hands to press upright to seated, keeping your chin toward your chest to support the neck. Reach your hands forward to the floor with palms flat, then lift into Table. Stretch the legs back, one at a time, curling the toes under on the floor to bring blood flow back through the knees. Transition to a seat or standing from here.

EXPERIENCE THE POSE
Feel every breath coax you toward relaxing your thighs, hips, back, and shoulders. Become mindful of sensations of lightness in the chest as you breathe.

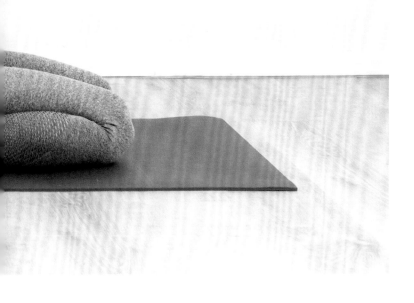

Supported Bridge
with two bolsters

RECOMMENDED TIME // 5–15 MINUTES

There's a benefit for everyone in this pose. It opens the lungs and chest, helps reverse forward head posture, and relieves fatigue as well as symptoms of mild depression and menopause, all while deeply quieting an overactive mind.

WHAT YOU NEED
- Mat
- Blanket
  » 1 basic fold
- Flat bolsters (2 or 1 flat and 1 round)
- Looped strap
- Eye pillow (optional)

PRECAUTIONS
Not recommended if you have a cold, sinus infection, indigestion, or uncontrolled hypertension. Do not practice if you are more than three months pregnant, or are not at least three months past the end of your pregnancy.

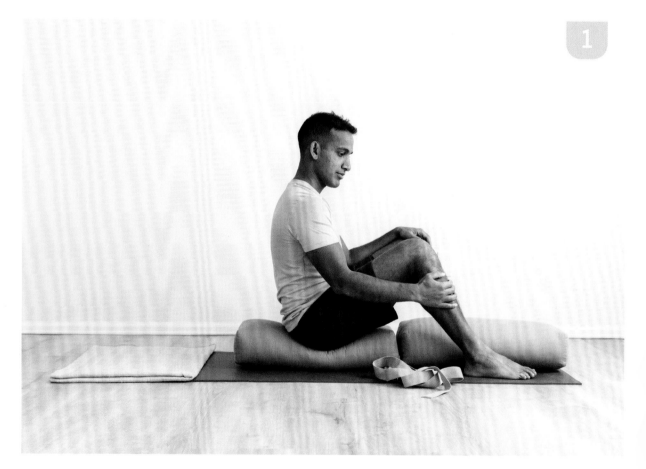

1

Position the bolsters lengthwise and end to end at the bottom half of the mat. Place the blanket at the top end of the mat, leaving about a hand's width of space between it and the bolsters. Sit on top of the bolster, facing away from the blanket with the strap off to the side.

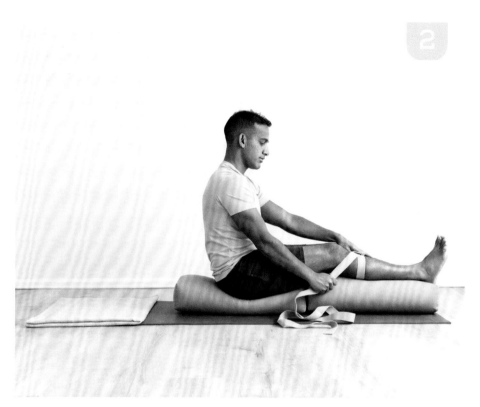

2

Slip the strap over your legs and tighten it around the middle of your calves. Extend your legs long, allowing your big toes to turn in while the heels relax slightly outward. *(If the heels extend beyond the bolsters, place blocks underneath them to bring them level with the bolsters.)*

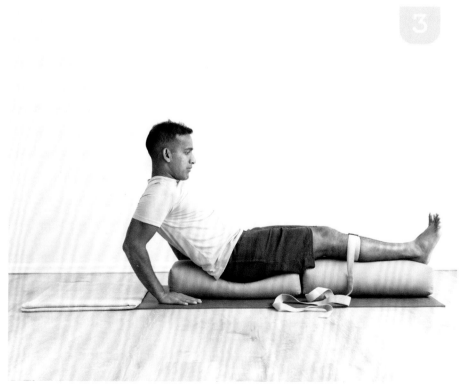

3

Using your hands for support, lower your upper body until your shoulders are resting on the floor and the back of your head is resting on the blanket. *(If you're unable to relax your shoulders, or your chin tips up significantly, replace the bolsters with folded blankets. If you experience low back discomfort, bend your knees, remove the strap, and set your feet wide to the sides of the bolster, then bring your knees together to touch.)*

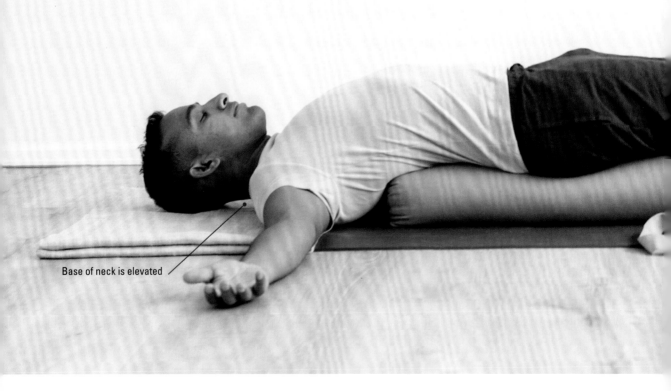

EXPERIENCE THE POSE
Let go of all facial tension
and soften your jaw. Become
receptive to the deep quality
of stillness, support, and quiet
that arrives in your mind as you
continue to hold this position.
Breathe naturally, feeling
your awareness recede
ever inward.

Base of neck is elevated

4

Apply the eye pillow or close your eyes, if it's comfortable. Reach your arms outward to a *T* shape, extending through the fingertips until you feel your shoulder blades widen, and then rotating the arms externally until your palms are facing up.

TRANSITION OUT: Returning at a snail's pace, bend your knees and place your feet on the bolster. Wiggle backward, sliding off the bolster far enough that your whole upper back meets the mat. Loosen the strap and then roll off the bolster to your side, resting your head on your arm. Stay for a few breaths, then slowly sit up.

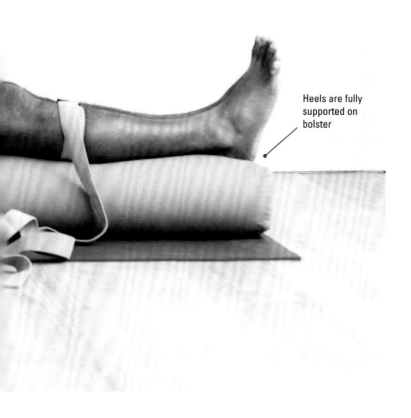

Heels are fully supported on bolster

Supported Bridge
with single bolster

RECOMMENDED TIME // 5-10 MINUTES

You'll release tension in the low back and feel rejuvenation in a heavy heart with this backbend that includes only a few props. This pose is also helpful for those who have tried Supported Bridge *with two bolsters* and found it aggravating for the lower back.

WHAT YOU NEED
- Mat
- Blanket
  » 1 basic fold
- Flat bolster
- Eye pillow (optional)

PRECAUTIONS
Not recommended if you have a cold, sinus infection, or indigestion. Do not practice if you are more than three months pregnant.

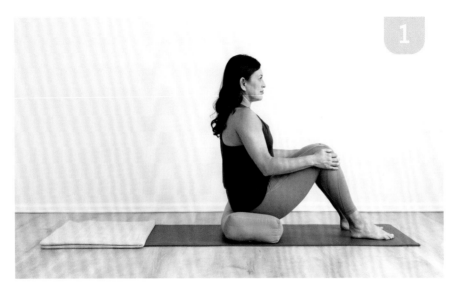

1

Position the bolster widthwise across the middle of the mat and place the basic-fold blanket at the top of the mat. Sit on top of the bolster with your buttocks and sacrum completely supported and your knees bent with your feet flat on the mat.

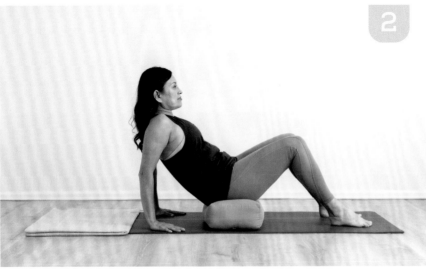

2

Place your hands by your sides and behind you for support, then carefully begin lowering your upper body down to the floor until your head is resting on the blanket.

EXPERIENCE THE POSE
Allow your shoulder blades to
drop heavily into the floor. Observe
any sensation in the abdomen as you
breathe fully in and out, and at a
smooth, slow pace, until you're
deeply relaxed, then allow the
breath to become natural and
simply be in the pose.

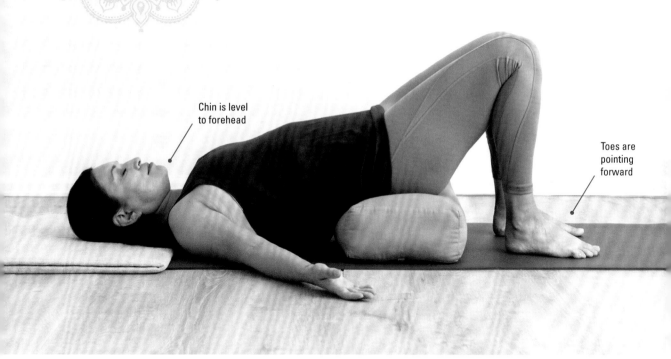

Chin is level
to forehead

Toes are
pointing
forward

Once you arrive at the floor, walk your heels back until they're
underneath your knees, making micro adjustments to the placement
of your feet until you feel like the legs are holding themselves up
with minimal effort. Apply the eye pillow or close your eyes, if it's
comfortable. Extend your arms outward and into a *V* shape, with
your palms facing up.

TRANSITION OUT: Press into the soles of the feet, lift the hips just slightly,
and push the bolster off the mat so you can rest your hips back to the floor. Lift
your feet and hug your knees toward your heart, cupping your knees with your
hands. Roll to one side and pause for a moment before pressing up to a seat.

Supported Wheel

RECOMMENDED TIME // 2–10 MINUTES

This backbend will help maintain a balanced, healthy posture in your whole spine. It's especially helpful for counteracting forward head posture and kyphosis, or roundback, which may result in shallow breathing, pain, headaches, and spinal degeneration.

WHAT YOU NEED
- Mat
- Blankets (3)
  » 3 basic fold
- Eye pillow (optional)

PRECAUTIONS
Do not practice if you are more than three months pregnant.

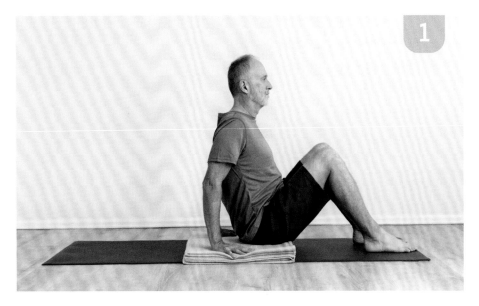

Stack the basic-fold blankets widthwise across the middle of the mat, with the neatly folded ends facing the top end of the mat. Sit on the edge of the blanket stack with your feet flat on the mat and at the bottom end of the mat, and your hands flat on the stack.

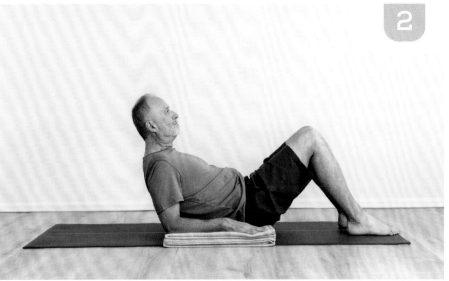

Keeping your knees bent and feet flat on the floor, use your forearms for support as you lower down until your upper body reaches the floor. Scoot forward or backward until you feel just the bottom tips of your shoulder blades touching the lip of the blanket stack. (If the position proves difficult, begin with fewer blankets until your body allows for more support.)

3

Walk the feet forward or backward until the soles feel evenly weighted on the mat. You may choose to keep the knees apart or support the legs by rotating the heels slightly outward and relaxing the knees together. Apply the eye pillow or close your eyes, if it's comfortable. Reach your arms out to a wide *T* or *V* shape until the shoulders feel relaxed. Turn the palms upward.

··

TRANSITION OUT: Exhale, separate your knees if needed, and gently push into your feet to slide your upper body backward until only your hips remain on the blankets. Take a few generous breaths in stillness, then roll to one side with your navel facing the floor. Use your hands to slowly sit up.

EXPERIENCE THE POSE
Expand the lungs fully with breath, then let go of all the air until you feel a natural emptiness in your abdomen. Do this twice more, releasing your body completely to gravity, then breathe naturally as you enter a softer state of being. Surrender all doing and become still.

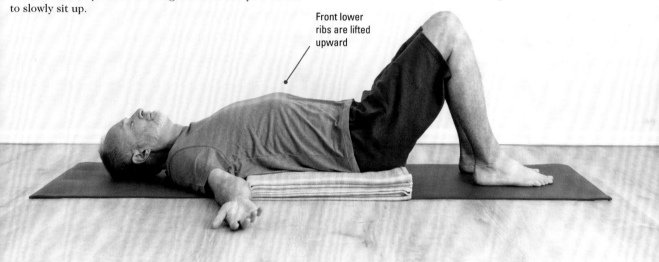

Front lower ribs are lifted upward

Variation

For more support in the lumbar spine as well as a deeper backbend, replace the basic–fold blankets with three rolled blankets placed next to one another across the middle of the mat, with the messy edges facing down. Sit with your back to the blankets, then practice the pose as instructed.

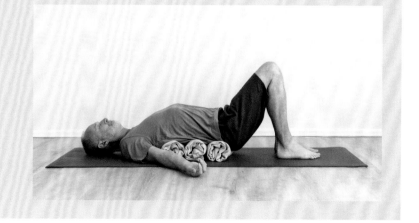

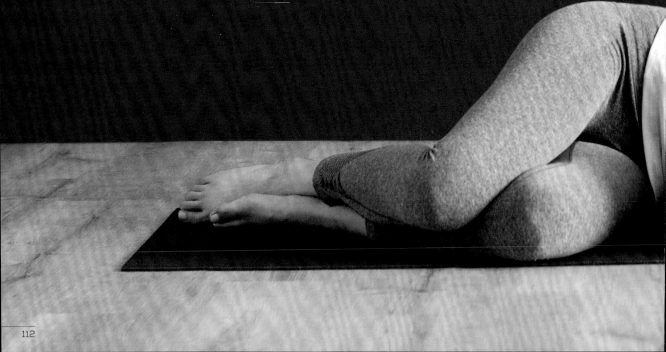

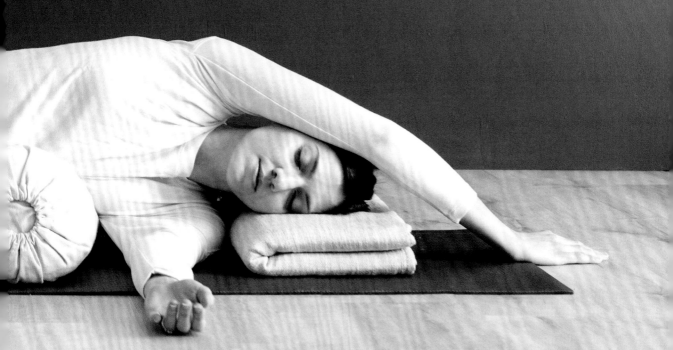

CHAPTER 4

Inversions, Twists, and Side Bends

Legs Up the Wall

RECOMMENDED TIME // 5-15 MINUTES

This gentle inversion relaxes the nervous system while encouraging the movement of lymphatic fluid and blood toward the upper body, which helps reduce fatigue and swelling in the legs, alleviate exhaustion, lower blood pressure, and calm a busy mind.

WHAT YOU NEED
- Mat
- Wall
- Blankets (2)
  » 1 square fold
  » 1 basic fold
- Looped strap (optional)
- Eye pillow (optional)

PRECAUTIONS
Consult with a healthcare professional if you have a hiatal hernia, heart issues, or eye issues. Do not practice if you are more than three months pregnant, menstruating, or at risk for miscarriage.

1

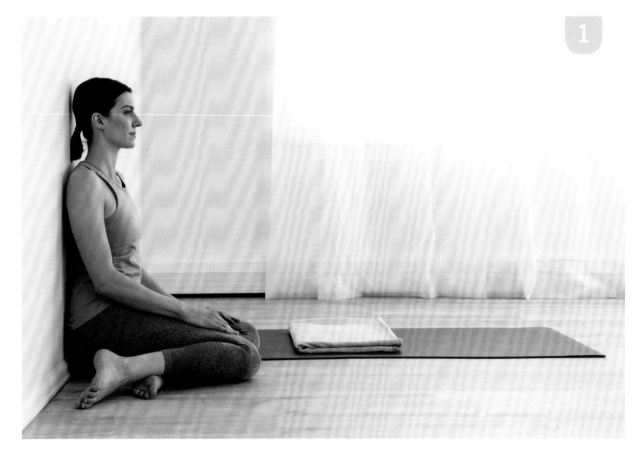

Align the mat to be perpendicular to an open wall. Place the basic-fold blanket at the bottom of the mat and against the wall, and the square-fold blanket in the middle of the mat. Sit on your left hip with your back against the wall and your legs tucked alongside your body. If using a strap, loop it and keep it nearby.

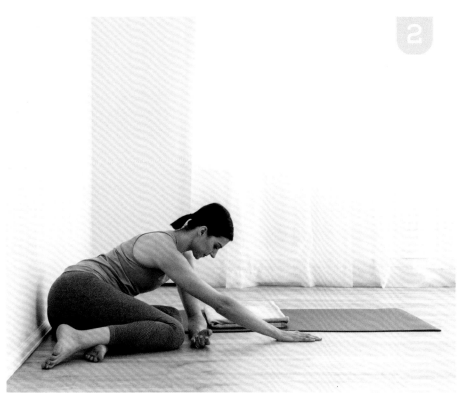

2 Lean forward while extending your left arm across your body and underneath your right arm until your forearm is flat on the floor.

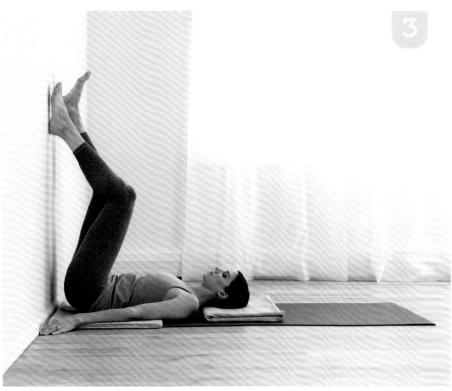

3 Use momentum to gently roll onto your back, while simultaneously swinging your legs up the wall. *(It's okay if your legs are not flush against the wall. If your hips are lifted or you feel tension in your hamstrings, scoot your hips away from the wall until they are fully grounded.)*

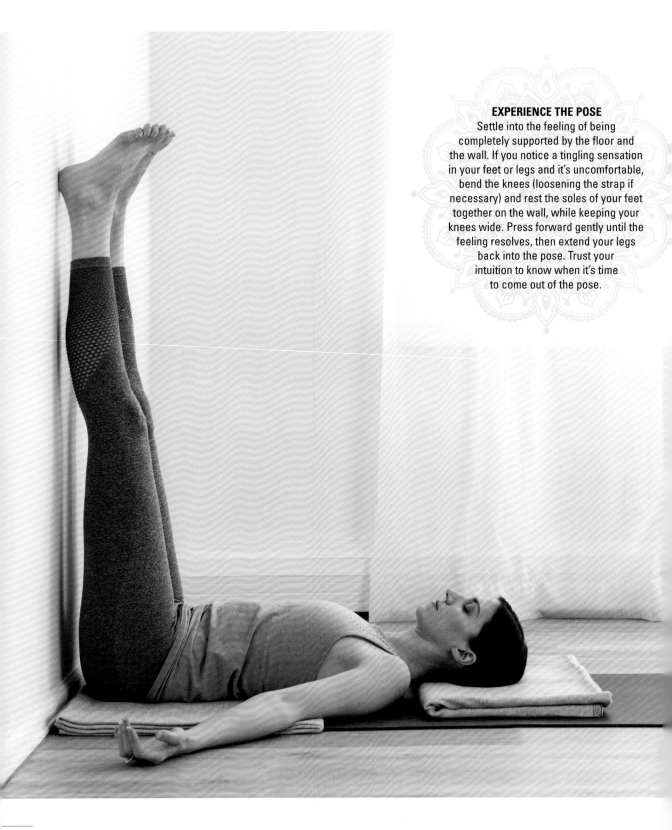

EXPERIENCE THE POSE
Settle into the feeling of being
completely supported by the floor and
the wall. If you notice a tingling sensation
in your feet or legs and it's uncomfortable,
bend the knees (loosening the strap if
necessary) and rest the soles of your feet
together on the wall, while keeping your
knees wide. Press forward gently until the
feeling resolves, then extend your legs
back into the pose. Trust your
intuition to know when it's time
to come out of the pose.

4 Adjust the blanket underneath the head so that the chin is slightly lower than the forehead. Apply the eye pillow or close your eyes, if it's comfortable, and rest your arms by your sides in a *V* shape with your palms facing up. *(If there's significant space between your legs and the wall, consider placing a bolster behind your legs for added comfort. If your legs splay outward or it feels like it's an effort to keep them up the wall, slide the looped strap over your feet and loosely cinch it around your upper shins, leaving about two fists' width of space between your calves.)*

TRANSITION OUT: Wiggle the toes and point and flex the feet, then slowly walk them down the wall and rest for a few easy breaths with your feet flat against the wall. Hug your legs toward your heart as you release your feet from the wall, then extend one arm overhead and slowly roll to that side, using your bicep to support your head. Take your time before pushing your hands into the floor and slowly sitting up.

Variation

This variation elevates your pelvis to create a gentle backbend and also stimulates digestion. You may also notice a sense of spaciousness in the upper chest and an ability to breathe deeper after practicing. To perform, place a flat bolster underneath your hips, about 4-6 inches (10-15cm) from the wall, and position your tailbone in the space between the wall and bolster. Avoid if you have indigestion. *(Add a rectangle-fold blanket under the upper spine and head if you experience pain.)*

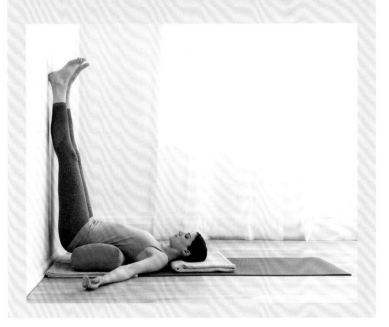

Legs Up the Wall
pregnancy variation

RECOMMENDED TIME // 5-10 MINUTES

This version of Legs Up the Wall is intended for pregnant women who are beyond their first trimester. It will help reduce swelling in the feet, ankles, and legs, while maintaining proper oxygen flow to the baby by elevating the mother's heart.

WHAT YOU NEED
- Mat
- Blankets (4)
  » 1 square fold
  » 3 rolled
- Blocks (3)
- Flat bolsters (2)
- Looped strap (optional)
- Eye pillow (optional)

PRECAUTIONS
Consult with your healthcare professional before practicing.

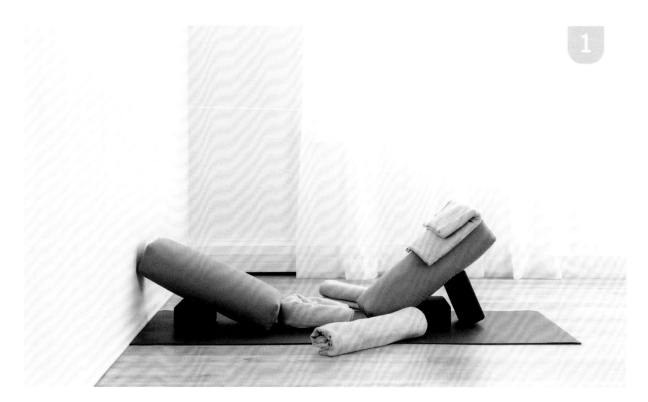

1

Position the mat so it's perpendicular to the wall. Tilt one bolster up against the wall and ramp it on a low block positioned about 6 inches (15cm) from the wall. Create a seat by making a circle out of a rolled blanket placed on the floor and next to the base of the bolster. Ramp the second bolster up a low block and a high block angled 45 degrees to the back of the bolster, and place the half-folded square-fold blanket at the high end of the bolster. Position two more rolled blankets along each side of the bolster ramp, each angled 45 degrees outward.

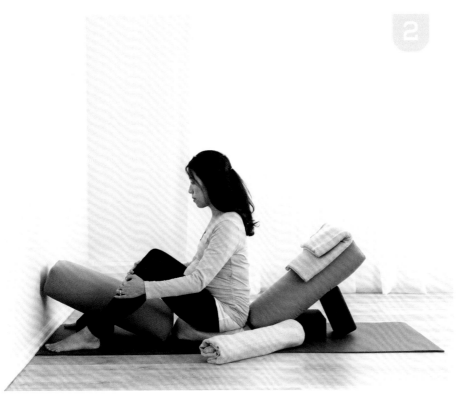

Sit on the seat so that the blanket wraps around the pelvis completely and the tailbone is centered in the blanket and lifted off the floor. Face the wall with your knees bent, and your feet placed flat on the mat and on the sides of the wall bolster. Adjust your distance from the wall until your legs are comfortable and your toes are nearly touching the wall.

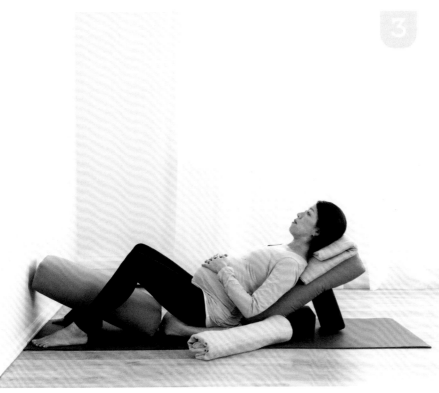

Using your hands for support, carefully recline to the ramped bolster behind you. Adjust the blanket underneath your neck and head so that they are both fully supported, and your chin is positioned lower than your forehead.

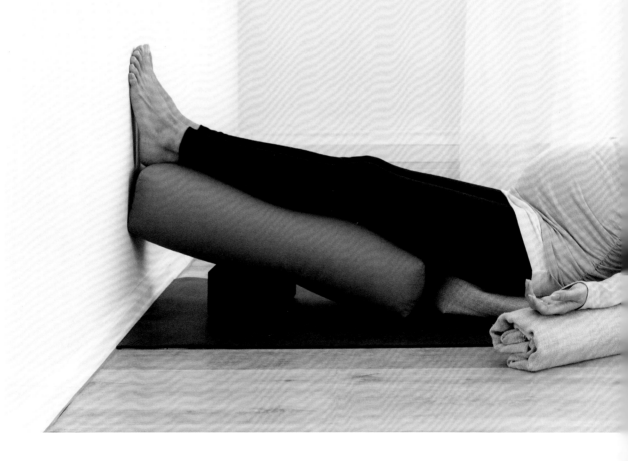

EXPERIENCE THE POSE
Give the weight of your body over to gravity, feeling the full support of the earth and the props rising up to meet you. Participate gently in your breath with progressively slower and smoother inhales and exhales, letting your body relax even more with every exhale.

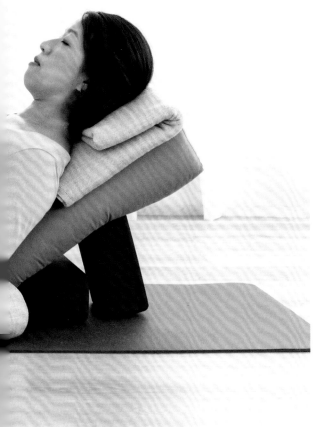

4 Step both feet onto the wall bolster, then walk them up the bolster until your heels are resting against the wall and your legs are fully extended. Apply the eye pillow or close your eyes, if it's comfortable. Relax your elbows and forearms onto the armrest blankets, with your palms facing up. *(If you can't keep your legs on the bolster without exerting significant effort, loosely cinch a strap around your upper shins to hold them together, making sure to keep a good amount of space between your knees and feet to make room for your abdomen. If your arms and hands aren't heavy and fully supported, add additional blankets.)*

TRANSITION OUT: When it's time to awaken from stillness, first become aware of the feeling of your feet and legs in relaxation, then make gentle movements with the toes. Slowly bend your knees (loosening the strap, if using) and step your feet to either side of the bolster. Stay present with your breath and take a moment to let the legs get used to the feeling of being on the floor. Move your right foot over the bolster to your left side. Lift the torso up by simultaneously pressing your palms into the mat and dropping your knees to the left, then exit the props and sit comfortably.

Side-Lying Stretch

RECOMMENDED TIME // 30 SECONDS TO 2 MINUTES

This pose will help you breathe easier by gently stretching the intercostal muscles between the ribs, which shrink and expand as you breathe. By actively stretching in this position, you are increasing your capacity for a fuller breath in the lungs, which can be helpful for treating respiratory conditions such as asthma.

WHAT YOU NEED
- Mat
- Flat bolster
- Round bolster
- Blankets (3, optional)

PRECAUTIONS
Consult with a healthcare professional if you have osteoporosis, a hiatal hernia, or you've had abdominal surgery. Do not practice if more than three months pregnant. If you experience back pain, try the supported version.

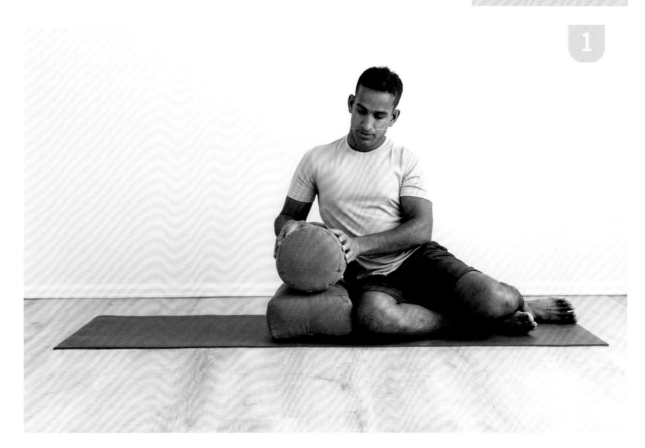

Position the flat bolster widthwise across the middle of the mat, then stack the round bolster on top. Sit on the mat with your right hip resting against the props and your hands holding the round bolster in position. *(Substitute 3 rectangle-fold blankets for the round bolster if the stack is too high for you.)*

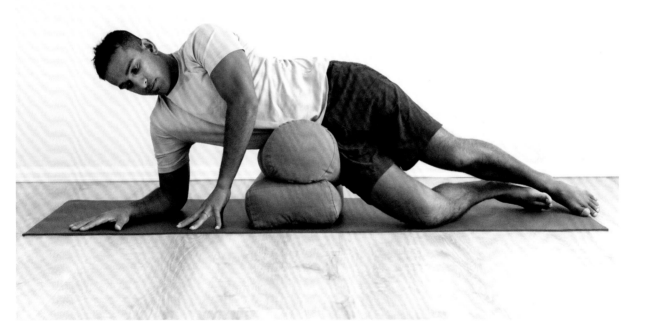

Lower your body down sideways so that your waist is fully supported by the bolsters and you sense equal weight hanging on both sides of the props. Make sure that you are fully side bending and not twisting in your upper or lower body, and that your hips and shoulders are vertically stacked. (If you experience any discomfort, slide up or down on the props until you feel fully supported.)

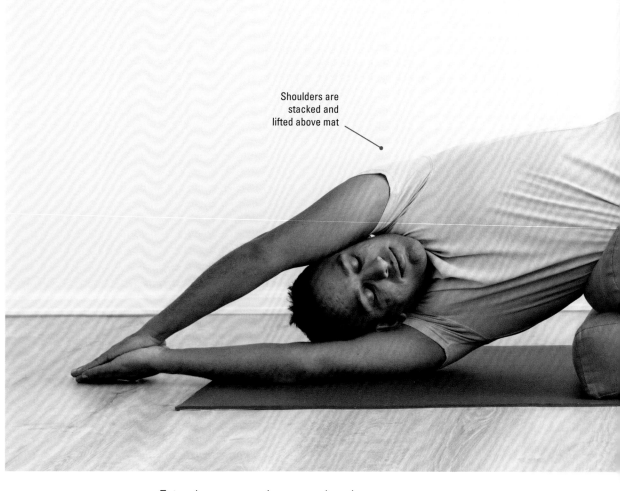

Shoulders are stacked and lifted above mat

Extend your arms above your head, resting your head on the bottom arm. Extend your legs like a pair of scissors while reaching through the heels to bring the top leg slightly forward and the bottom leg slightly back. Relax the weight of the legs onto the floor, but remain lightly active in your heels to keep the legs straight.

TRANSITION OUT: Bend your knees and let your hips drop to the mat as you bend your elbows toward the bolsters. Press into your palms to sit up. Pause for a breath before repeating the pose on the opposite side.

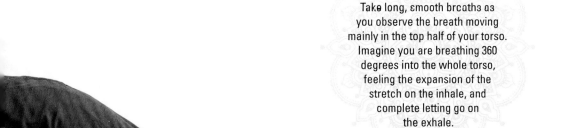

EXPERIENCE THE POSE
Take long, smooth breaths as
you observe the breath moving
mainly in the top half of your torso.
Imagine you are breathing 360
degrees into the whole torso,
feeling the expansion of the
stretch on the inhale, and
complete letting go on
the exhale.

Variation

Grasp your top wrist
with your bottom
hand and lightly pull
it overhead to create
even more opening
in the rib cage.

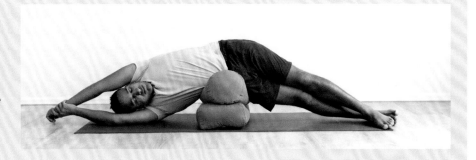

Supported Side-Lying Stretch

RECOMMENDED TIME // 3 MINUTES PER SIDE

This passive version of Side-Lying Stretch features all the same benefits as the unsupported version. You'll experience enhanced breathing, and lying on the left side assists the function of your gallbladder and liver, while lying on the right side benefits the stomach and spleen.

WHAT YOU NEED
- Mat
- Blankets (2–3)
  » 2 double-square fold
  » 1 rolled (optional)
- Round bolster
- Flat bolster

PRECAUTIONS
Consult with a healthcare professional if you have osteoporosis, a hiatal hernia, or you've had abdominal surgery. Do not practice if more than three months pregnant.

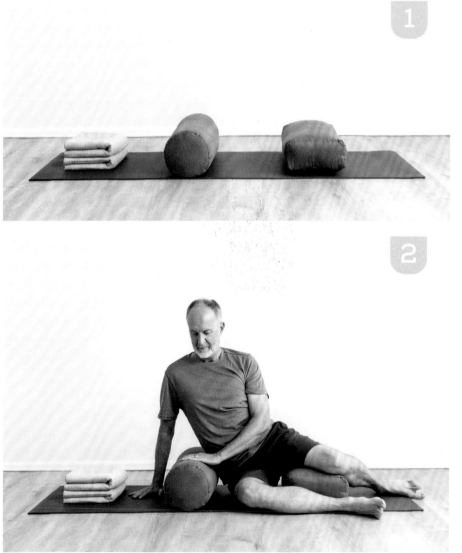

1 Stack the two double-square-fold blankets at the top of the mat. Position the round bolster widthwise about 12 inches (30cm) from the double-square-fold blankets, then position the flat bolster about 12 inches (30cm) from the round bolster. If using, place the optional rolled blanket beside the mat but within reach.

2 Sit on your right hip between the round and flat bolsters. Arrange your right knee and calf on the mat and in front of the flat bolster, and place your left knee on top of the bolster. Your right knee should extend from your hip at a 90-degree angle, while your left knee should be extended at a 45-degree angle. Hold the round bolster against your waist with your left hand and press your right palm into the floor in the space between the blankets and round bolster.

3

Inhale and lengthen your whole right side up and away from the round bolster, then exhale and lower your torso down sideways as you reach your right forearm forward until your right shoulder touches the floor and the right side of your face is supported by the blankets. Extend your left arm over your head, resting your left bicep on your head and softening the wrist and fingers to the floor. Close your eyes, if it's comfortable.

(If you experience discomfort in your arms or shoulders, hug the optional rolled blanket to your chest with your elbow on the round bolster.)

TRANSITION OUT: Return your left hand to the floor and in front of your face. Exhale and use gentle effort to press down into the palm to rise up sideways and away from the props. Turn away from the round bolster, lifting your knees up, then dropping them down to your left. Transition to your opposite hip and repeat the pose.

EXPERIENCE THE POSE

Release any tension in the upper body and the legs, feeling your spine flowing like a wave over the props. Breathe smoothly and steadily.

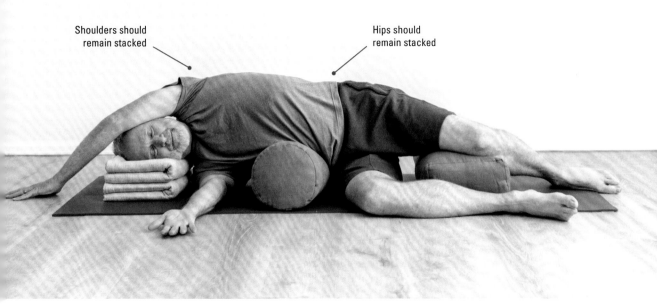

Shoulders should remain stacked

Hips should remain stacked

Variation

If it's uncomfortable to extend your arm above your head, you can rest it on the side of your body, with your hand resting on your hip.

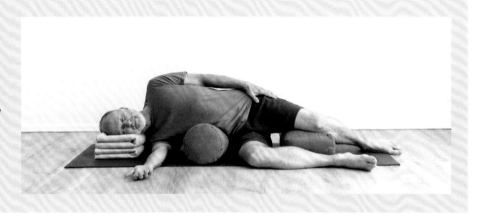

Supported Spinal Twist

RECOMMENDED TIME // 1–3 MINUTES PER SIDE
(if pregnant, practice for 30–90 seconds per side)

This gentle twist relieves tension between the shoulder blades and enhances breathing by opening the intercostals, the small muscles between the ribs that participate in torso rotation. This pose can also influence the sternocleidomastoid, a muscle that runs along each side of the neck and when tight can contribute to headaches, migraines, and neck pain.

WHAT YOU NEED
- Mat
- Blankets (1–2)
  » double-square fold
  » rectangle fold (optional)
- Flat bolster

PRECAUTIONS
Follow the Safe Practice Guidelines (p. 28) if you have back pain or acute sacroiliac issues. If you're pregnant, sit farther away from the bolster to accommodate your abdomen, and focus more on twisting from your upper chest rather than from your belly.

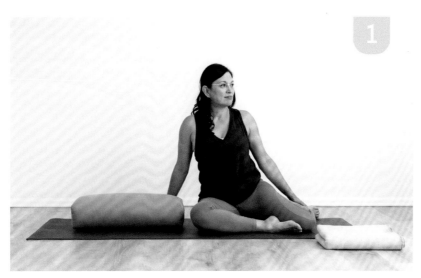

1 Position the flat bolster lengthwise along the top half of the mat. Place the double-square-fold blanket next to the mat and within reach. Sit sideways on your right hip and near the end of the bolster, with your knees bent and legs dropped into a pinwheel shape. *(If you need extra support for your head, place the optional rectangle-fold blanket lengthwise on the bolster.)*

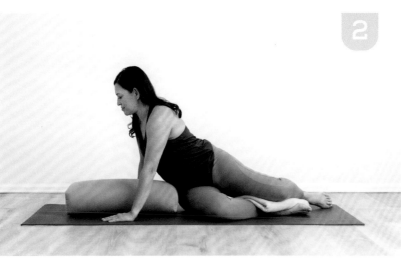

2 Nestle your left calf muscle on top of your right foot. Adjust your legs until comfortable, then place the double-square-fold blanket between your left knee and right ankle. Place your palms flat along the sides of the mat, then twist your upper body and navel over the middle of the bolster. Press down into your palms, inhale, and lengthen the front of your body upward, then exhale and slowly begin to lower your torso down to the bolster.

3

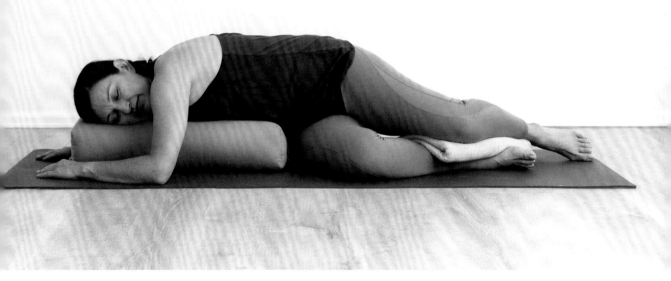

Turn your right cheek to the bolster as you arrive
at the bolster. Slide your forearms forward while
bending your elbows outward until your palms are
flat on the ground and in front of the bolster. Close
your eyes, if it's comfortable.

TRANSITION OUT: Bend your elbows and slide your
palms back to your shoulders. Inhale and push through
your hands to gently rise up to seated while simultaneously
unwinding the twist. Turn to the opposite side and repeat
the pose with your left hip positioned against the bolster.

Supported Supine Spinal Twist

RECOMMENDED TIME // 2–3 MINUTES

This twist is a go-to favorite of mine for relaxing tension in the chest, shoulders, and back. As an added benefit, by twisting to the right first and then to the left, this posture stimulates digestion and encourages healthy elimination.

WHAT YOU NEED
- Mat
- Blankets (3)
  » 1 double-rectangle fold
  » 1 rectangle fold
  » 1 square fold
- Flat bolster

PRECAUTIONS
Do not practice if you have osteoporosis. Consult with a healthcare professional if you have acute sacroiliac issues or have had abdominal surgery. Do not practice if you are more than three months pregnant.

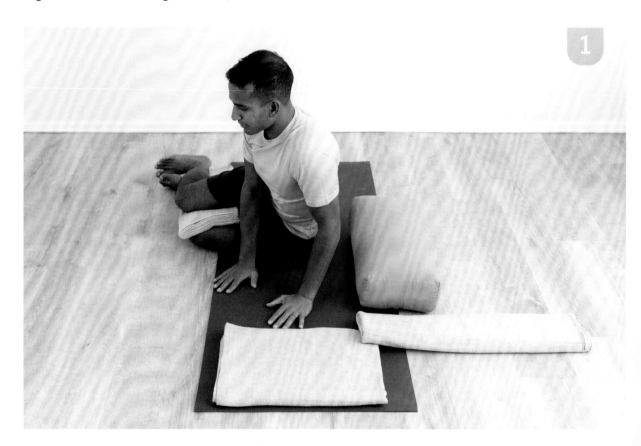

1

Place the square-fold blanket across the top end of the mat, then extend the double-rectangle-fold blanket out from the square-fold blanket and off the side of the mat. Position the flat bolster lengthwise along the side of the mat. Sit on your left hip in the middle of the mat, with your legs stacked and the rectangle-fold blanket sandwiched between your legs from the knees to the ankles. (If you experience pain in your sacrum area, increase the thickness of the blanket between your knees.)

Use your hands to lower down onto your left side as you extend your left arm forward with your palm facing up and then reach your right arm behind you to snug the bolster up against your back, so it's positioned just beneath your armpit, leaving some space behind your shoulder.

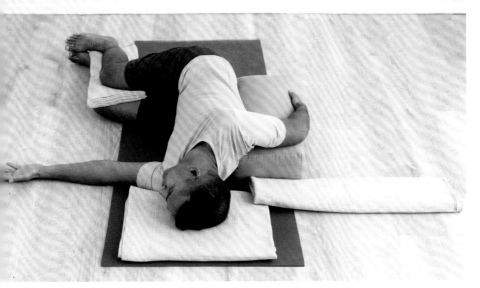

Adjust the blanket under your head and neck until they feel at ease and your left shoulder is in line with your left hip. Return your right hand to meet your left. Arrange your knees 90 degrees from your hips, with your feet stacked directly beneath your knees.

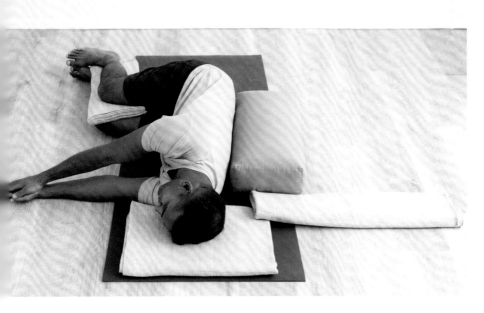

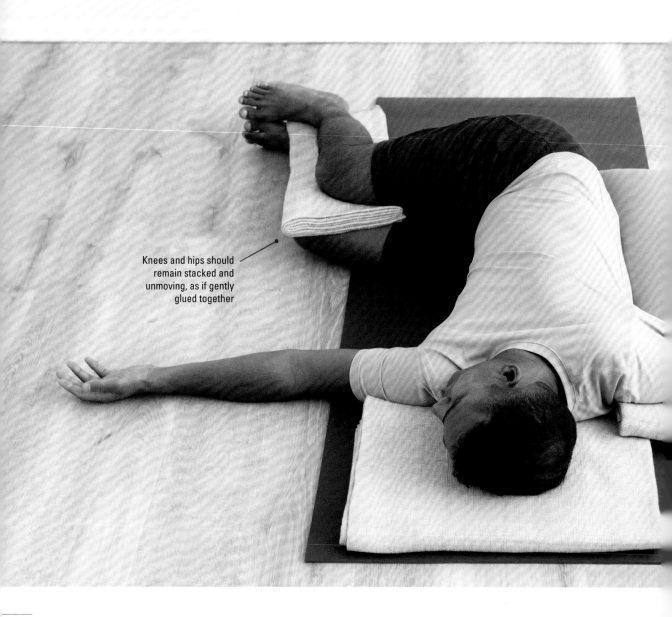

Knees and hips should remain stacked and unmoving, as if gently glued together

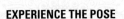

EXPERIENCE THE POSE
Feel the stable support of the bolster at your back as your arms and chest expand. Just breathe smoothly.

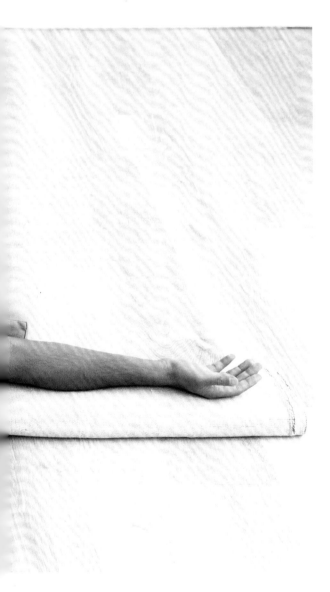

Exhale as you arc your right arm behind you while gently twisting open from the upper body. Encourage a gentle openness in the shoulders and front of the chest by opening and closing the right arm back and forth 3-5 times while following your fingers with your gaze, then resting in stillness with the right arm remaining open in the twist. Your gaze may be left, up, or right, whichever position is the most pleasant. Close your eyes, if it's comfortable. *(If you experience tingling or numbness in the fingers, lower the arms down to an angle where the feeling is resolved.)*

TRANSITION OUT: Inhale as you raise your right arm up, then exhale as you close it on top of the left. Keeping the blanket squeezed between your legs, roll onto your back, pushing aside the bolster if necessary. Pressing the knees gently together with feet wide and flat on the mat, take three easy breaths. Feel both shoulder blades heavy on the ground. Move the bolster over to the left side of the mat, roll to your right hip, and repeat the pose on this side.

Variation

This twist may also be practiced with the bolster placed horizontally across the mat and your hips stacked on the bolster. In this case, your knees will be lower to the floor and below the bolster as your upper body opens in the twist. You may experience a spacious sense of expansion throughout the entire rib cage, waist, and hip region, plus an ability to breathe more deeply. If your low back is aggravated in the twist, lower the height of the hips by using a double-rectangle-fold blanket instead.

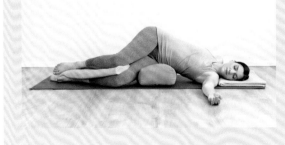

Upward-Facing Forward Bend

RECOMMENDED TIME // 2–5 MINUTES

The inverted leg position of this pose offers a gentle squeeze to the abdominal organs, encouraging blood flow to support healthy function. In addition to providing relief for tired legs, the pose may also improve symptoms in women who have a prolapsed uterus or bladder. (Be sure to wait at least two hours after eating before practicing this pose.)

WHAT YOU NEED
- Mat
- Flat bolster
- Eye pillow (optional)

PRECAUTIONS
Do not practice if you have a cold or sinus infection, indigestion, or a hiatal hernia. Additionally, do not practice if you are menstruating, are more than three months pregnant, or are not at least three months past the end of your pregnancy.

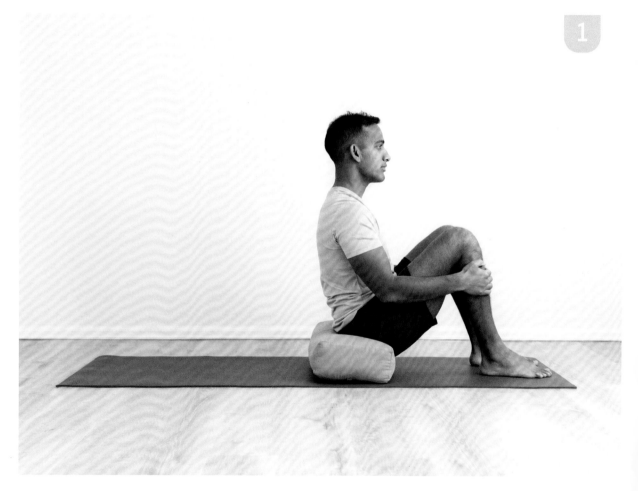

1

Place the flat bolster widthwise across the middle of the mat. Sit in the middle of the bolster with your feet flat at the bottom edge of the mat.

2 Using your hands for support, slowly begin to lower your upper body down until your shoulders and head are resting on the mat. The sacrum and lower back should be fully supported and heavy on the bolster.

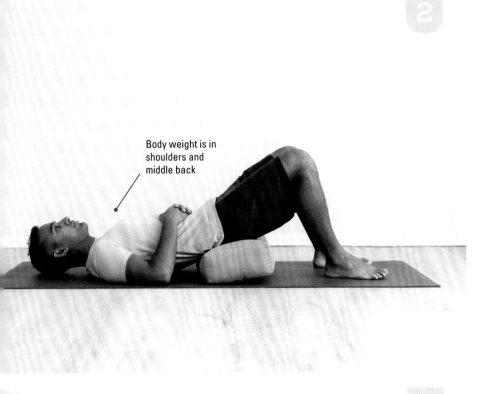

Body weight is in shoulders and middle back

3 Widen your arms on the floor for support as you exhale and bend your knees one at a time toward your chest.

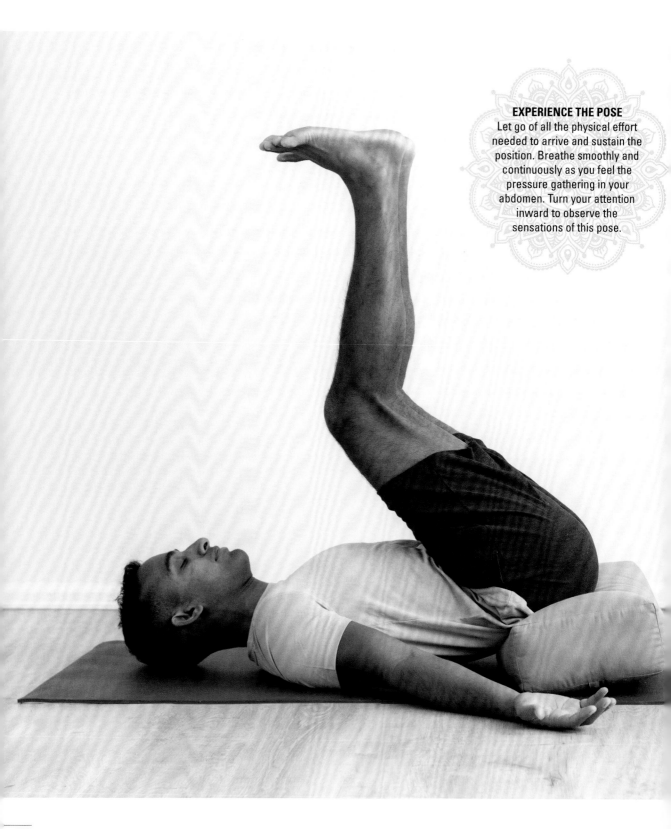

EXPERIENCE THE POSE
Let go of all the physical effort needed to arrive and sustain the position. Breathe smoothly and continuously as you feel the pressure gathering in your abdomen. Turn your attention inward to observe the sensations of this pose.

4 Extend your legs upward and toward your head, allowing them to float above your body without effort. Apply the eye pillow or close your eyes, if it's comfortable, and extend your arms in a *V* shape with your palms facing up.

....

TRANSITION OUT: Remove the eye pillow, if using. Exhale and bend your knees until your feet are resting on the floor in front of the bolster. Push into your heels to slide your upper body off the bolster until the bolster is underneath your knees. Breathe easily, observing the spaciousness in your abdomen.

Variation

If your hamstrings feel uncomfortably stretched in this pose, place a rolled blanket between your thighs and abdomen. You can adjust the thickness of the blanket roll or bend your knees as much as needed until your legs feel at ease. If you're still experiencing discomfort, replace the bolster with 1–2 rectangle-fold blankets.

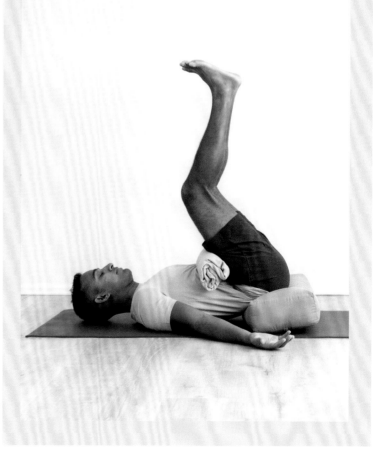

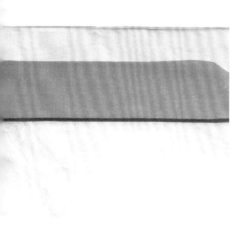

Stonehenge

RECOMMENDED TIME // 10–20 MINUTES

Named after its resemblance to the iconic, historical monument, this position bestows its own sense of deep presence and rejuvenating power when practiced mindfully. It's also a standout posture for alleviating low back pain.

WHAT YOU NEED
- Mat
- Blankets (2–3)
  » 1 basic fold
  » 1 headrest
  » 1 double-rectangle fold (optional)
- Blocks (2)
- Flat bolster
- Looped strap (optional)
- Eye pillow (optional)

PRECAUTIONS
If you are more than three months pregnant, practice the pregnancy version instead.

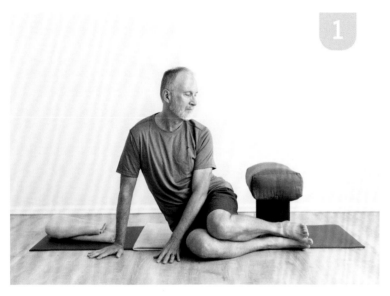

1 Place two high blocks parallel to one another at the bottom third of the mat with about two fists' width of space between them, then stack the bolster on top of the blocks. Place the basic-fold blanket widthwise across the middle of the mat, then position the headrest blanket at the top end of the mat. Sit on your right hip on the blanket, with your legs stacked and hands flat on the floor.

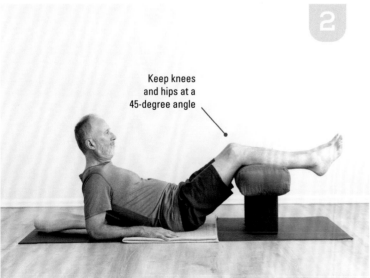

Keep knees and hips at a 45-degree angle

2 Swing your legs up and on top of the bolster, hooking the backs of your knees onto the edge of the bolster while simultaneously lowering back onto your forearms. *(If your legs splay open or will not relax without effort, loop a loose strap around your upper thighs to gently hold your legs in place.)*

3

Use your hands for support as you lower your upper body down to the mat. Adjust the headrest blanket so that your forehead is slightly higher than your chin. Apply the eye pillow or close your eyes, if it's comfortable, and extend your arms into a wide *V* shape with your palms facing up. *(If your lower back is significantly arched, add a double-rectangle-fold blanket on top of the bolster. Then lift your hips slightly, tilt your tailbone up, and lower the hips down.)*

TRANSITION OUT:
Sense your toes with your inner awareness, then begin to wiggle them and gently move your ankles. Let this action ripple into the pulling of your knees toward your heart while lifting your legs away from the bolster. Reach one arm overhead and roll to one side, resting your head on your bicep. Take your time before slowly sitting up.

EXPERIENCE THE POSE
Steep yourself in the pleasant dual sensations of lightness in the legs and complete grounded support in the upper body. Enter into stillness by noticing your gentle breath and then releasing all effort, giving yourself permission to do nothing but relax.

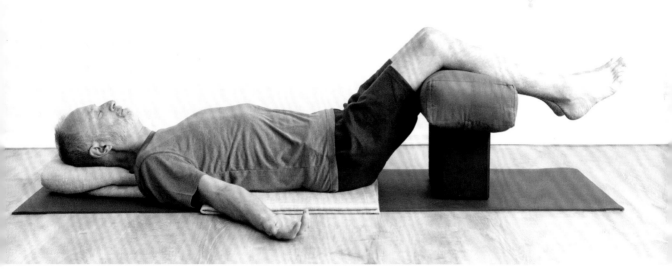

Variation

For extra support and back pain relief, try legs up a chair with your knees hovering above your hips. Pad the top of the chair with one square-fold blanket, then practice the pose as instructed. *(You can use low chairs or couches if you don't have a yoga chair, just make sure your feet are either level with or lower than your knees.)*

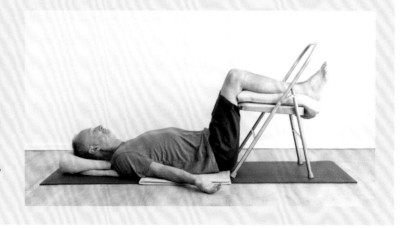

Stonehenge
pregnancy variation

RECOMMENDED TIME // 10-20 MINUTES

This pregnancy variation of Stonehenge is intended for women who are more than three months pregnant. It can provide relief from fluid buildup and swelling in the legs and feet, while still keeping baby safe.

WHAT YOU NEED
- Mat
- Blankets (6)
  » 2 rolled
  » 2 double-rectangle fold
  » 1 basic fold
  » 1 square fold
- Blocks (2)
- Flat bolster
- Round bolster
- Eye pillow (optional)

PRECAUTIONS
Consult with your healthcare professional before practicing.

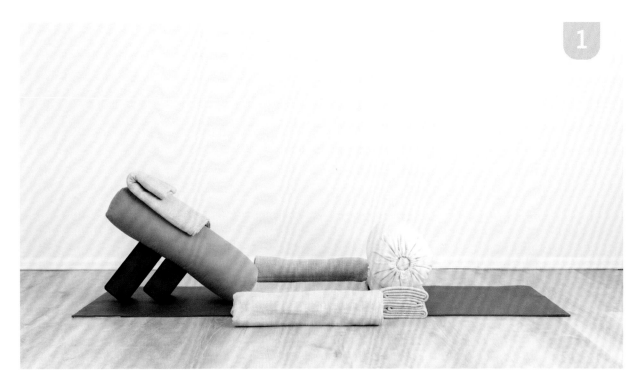

1

Stack the double-rectangle-fold blankets widthwise at the bottom third of the mat, then stack the round bolster on top. Place the basic-fold blanket in the middle of the mat, then place the two rolled blankets next to the basic-fold blanket. Set two blocks, one high and one medium, at the top of the mat, then ramp the bolster up the angled blocks. Stack the square-fold blanket, folded down by one-third, at the top of the bolster.

2

Sit on the blanket with your back against the flat bolster, then swing your legs up and over the round bolster while hooking the backs of your knees onto the bolster's edge.

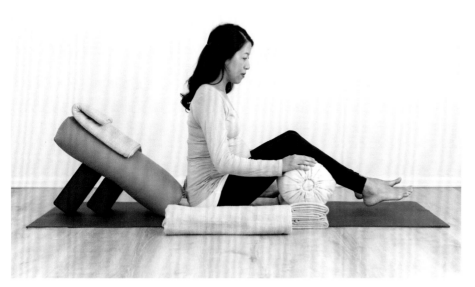

3

Use your hands for support as you lower your upper body down to the bolster. Adjust the square-fold blanket so that your forehead is slightly higher than your chin, then apply the eye pillow or close your eyes, if it's comfortable. *(If you experience any discomfort, you can add additional blankets underneath your tailbone, arms, or head.)*

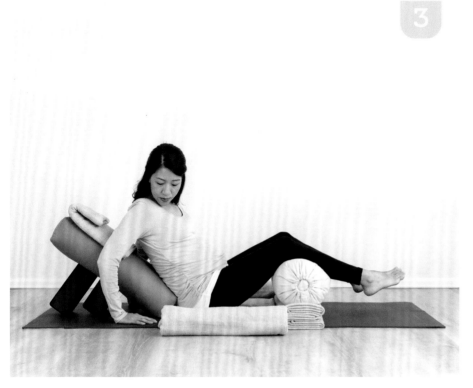

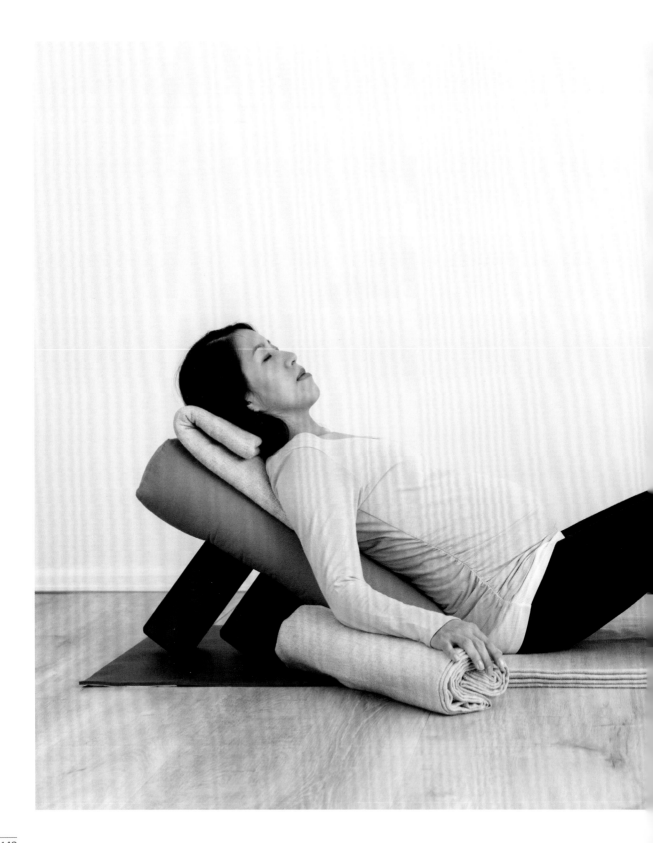

Extend your arms out onto the blankets positioned at your sides so that your elbows and wrists are completely supported by the blankets. Your palms may face down or up. Before arriving in stillness, make any adjustments to ensure this position is completely comfortable.

TRANSITION OUT: Exhale and bend your knees one at a time, then place your feet on top of the round bolster, and roll it away from you just far enough that your feet are firmly on the mat with your knees wide and in front of the blanket stack. Sit up by simultaneously pressing your palms into the floor and dropping your knees to the left, using just enough momentum to press your upper body to a seat.

EXPERIENCE THE POSE
Connect with the effortlessness arriving in your feet and legs and with the gentle breath moving in and out of your body.

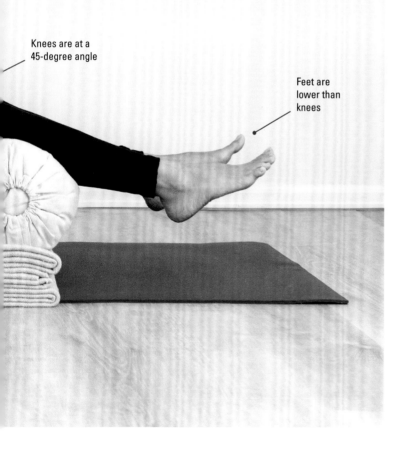

Knees are at a 45-degree angle

Feet are lower than knees

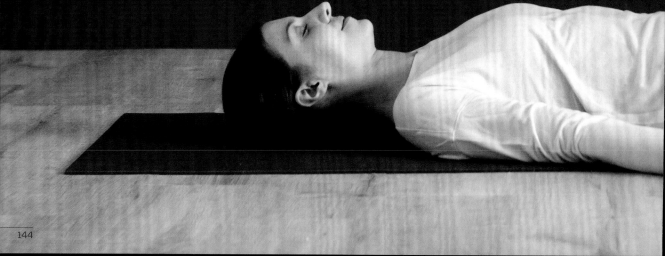

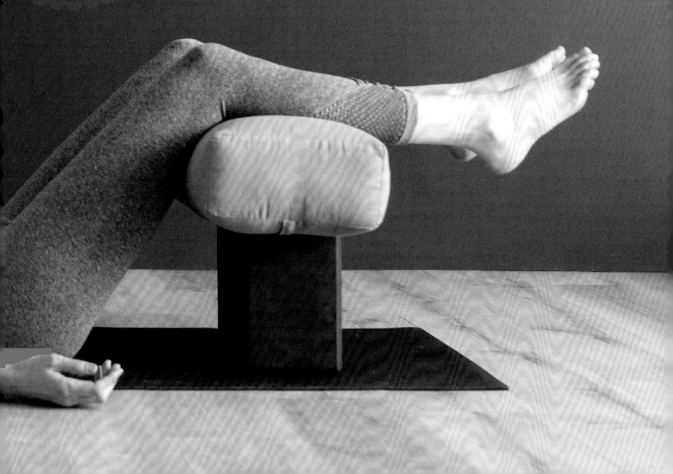

CHAPTER 5

Restorative Sequences

Minimal Props

TOTAL TIME // 40 MINUTES

WHAT YOU NEED
- Timer
- Mat
- Wall
- Chair
- Pillow (optional)

This sequence uses just a few props; it's great when you're traveling, or you just desire a more simplistic practice. We often stop ourselves from doing new things because we don't feel prepared. This practice is a reminder that all you need is yourself.

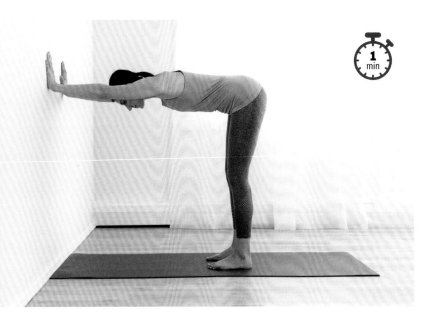

1. Place the mat for **Half-Dog at Wall (p. 44)** and come into the pose. Take voluminous breaths into the entire rib cage and abdomen—front, sides and back—as you firmly connect your palms to the wall and the soles of your feet to the floor.

TRANSITION: Inhale, place your hands on your hips, then contract your thigh muscles and slowly rise to standing.

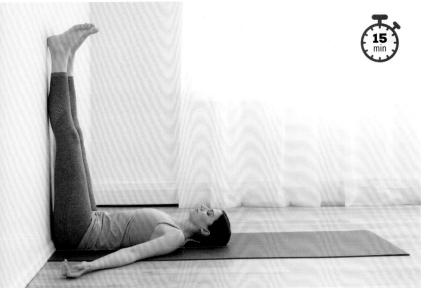

2. Move to the floor and come into **Legs Up the Wall (p. 114)**. Count down from 5 to 1 as you practice **Lengthen the Exhale (p. 32)** with quiet breath. Feel the air sweep effortlessly through the nasal passages, then release all effort with the breath and become aware of how sensations of heaviness and lethargy are draining from your body.

TRANSITION: Exhale, then walk your feet down the wall and roll to one side. Rest for a few breaths. Take your time to sit up.

3. Sit in front of a chair (perhaps adding a pillow for softness) and lean forward into **Supported Seated Forward Bend** *with chair* **(variation) (p. 77)**. Make no effort or sound with your breath so that your mind may transition into stillness like a rippling pool of water smoothing toward a still, reflective surface. Stay for 2 minutes, then change the cross of your legs and continue the pose for 2 minutes more.

....

TRANSITION: Inhale and slowly lift your torso upright.

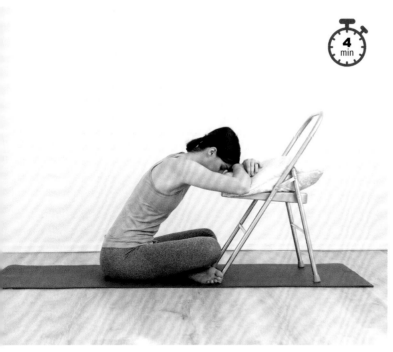

4. Recline to your back and swing your legs up on the chair to come into **Stonehenge (variation) (p. 139)**. Visualize through full, slow exhalations that all obligations, tasks, and worries that keep you from relaxing are dissolving into the earth. Do this without effort until you feel content, then release the visual and just breathe naturally.

....

TRANSITION: Exhale as you bend your knees toward your heart and roll to one side. Sit up and move away from the chair.

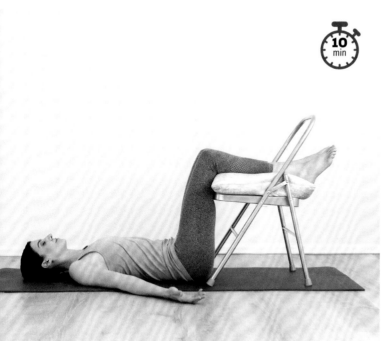

5. Lie down on your back for **Basic Relaxation Pose (p. 37)**. Practice **Mindful Yawning (p. 31)** to deepen your experience of relaxation, then just relax, knowing there is nothing left to do—only to be.

Relieving Lower Back Pain

TOTAL TIME // 45 MINUTES

Many factors can contribute to back pain, so consider this one healing tool in your journey. Before you begin, visualize an activity you used to enjoy when you were pain-free, then close your eyes and see yourself doing that activity now, but without pain. Begin with this hopeful energy.

WHAT YOU NEED
- Timer
- Mat
- Chair
- Blankets (4)
- Block
- Flat bolster
- Round bolster
- Looped strap
- Hand towel
- Eye pillow (optional)

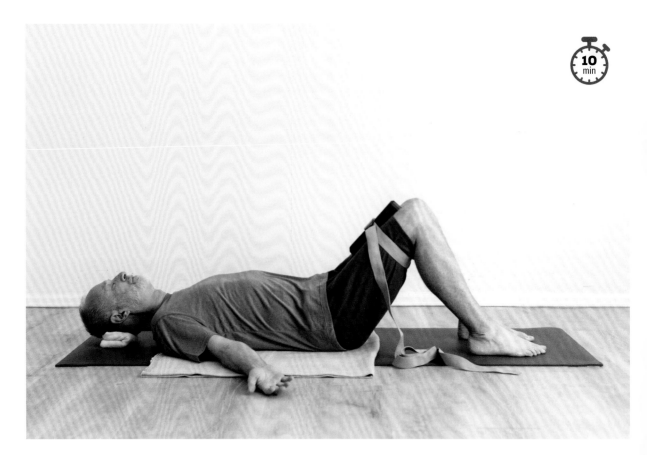

10 min

1. Place the props for **Constructive Rest Position (p. 80)** and come into the pose. Once you arrive, tell your lower back muscles that it's okay to let go. Practice **Longer, Smoother, Softer Breathing (p. 32)** for as long as you can stay present with it, then just breathe naturally.

TRANSITION: Remove the props from your legs, then extend your legs long on the floor. Bend your knees and roll to one side. Take your time to sit up.

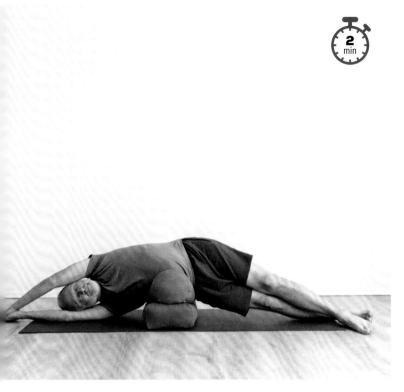

2. Place the props for **Side-Lying Stretch (p. 122)** and lower down onto your right side and into the pose, allowing your waist to release heavily toward the floor. Continue with **Longer, Smoother, Softer Breathing (p. 32)**, feeling as though you are expanding gently into the sides of the ribs on the inhale and releasing completely on the exhale. Hold for 1 minute, then lift your chest up sideways and allow your hips to drop to the mat. Turn away from the bolster and move to the opposite hip to repeat the pose on the other side for 1 minute.

TRANSITION: Drop your hip to the floor as you lift up sideways to seated.

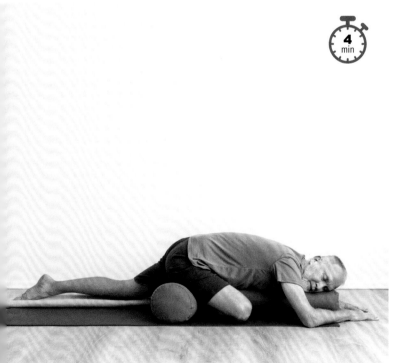

3. Place the props for **Supported Pigeon (p. 64)** and lower into the pose with your right foot forward. Before you lower your chest fully, bend your back leg inward and hold onto it with your left hand, gently stretching the quadriceps muscles for five calm breaths, then release the foot and fully enter the pose. Hold for 2 minutes, breathing naturally, then rise to Table. Extend the right leg long behind you for a few breaths, with your toes tucked on the mat. Move the blanket to the other side of the mat and repeat the pose on the opposite side for 2 minutes.

TRANSITION: Exhale and rise back to Table to stretch the left leg backward until you feel at ease in the knees and hips.

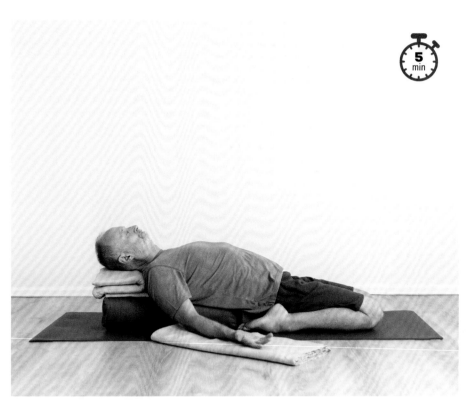

4. Place the props for **Supported Reclining Hero (p. 96)** and recline back into the pose. Before entering complete stillness, breathe in and curl your fingers in toward your palms, then breathe out and release your fingers, letting go of tension wherever you may feel it in your body. Do this five times, then breathe naturally and become still. Let any areas with muscle tension know that it's okay to let go.

TRANSITION: Exhale and rise to Table, stretching your legs back one at a time, then face the bolster to set up for the next pose.

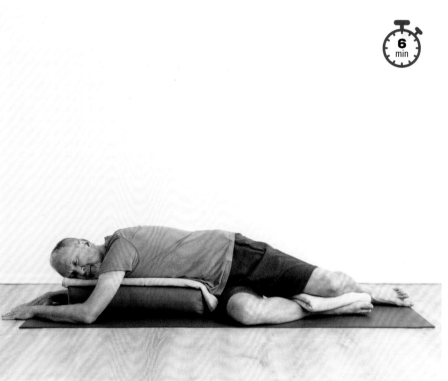

5. Place the props for **Supported Spinal Twist (p. 128)** and enter the pose on your right hip. Allow the breath to quiet and become natural without any modifications. Hold for 3 minutes, then, moving slowly, rise to seated as you unwind the twist. Keep your knees hugged together as you turn to the opposite side to repeat the pose for 3 minutes.

TRANSITION: Remove the blanket from your knees, then slowly sit up.

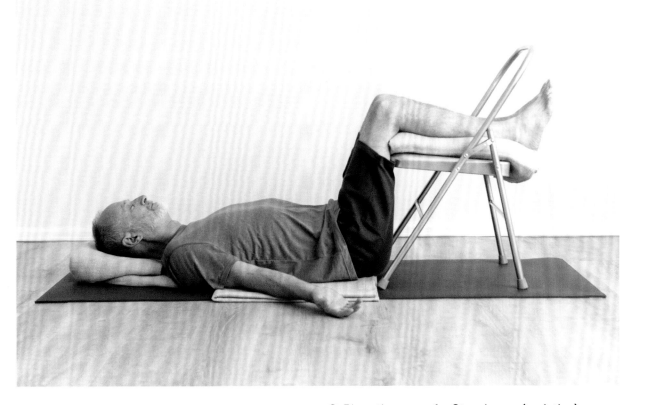

6. Place the props for **Stonehenge (variation) (p. 139)** and come into the pose. Release all effort in the abdomen as you breathe naturally.

....

TRANSITION: Exhaling, carefully bend your knees in toward your chest, scooting backward if needed, and drop your knees to one side. Rest there for a couple rounds of breath, then slowly sit up.

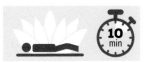

7. Place the props for **Basic Relaxation Pose (p. 37)** and come into the pose. Recall the intention you began this practice with and imagine yourself again doing an activity you love without pain. Plant this feeling like a seed into your heart as you relax all effort and rest in stillness.

Easing Head, Neck, and Shoulder Tension

WHAT YOU NEED
- Timer
- Mat
- Blankets (3)
- Blocks (2)
- Flat bolsters (2)
- Round bolster
- Looped strap
- Eye pillow (optional)

TOTAL TIME // 35 MINUTES

Pain and tension are signals from the brain and body to get you to pay attention and make a change. Instead of pushing through tension—ignoring or suppressing it—practice this sequence to reconnect to the part of you that is free from physical, mental, and emotional agitation.

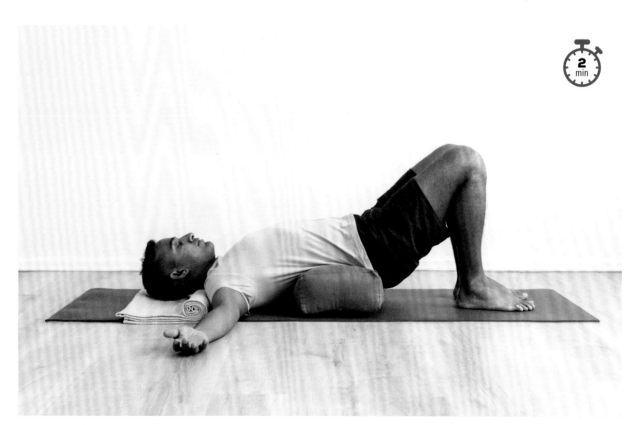

🕑 **2 min**

1. Place the props for **Simple Supported Backbend (p. 82)** and come into the pose. Scan through your body and breathe into any areas that feel constricted, mentally softening those areas as you exhale.

. . . .

TRANSITION: Slide your upper body backward off the bolster, then push the bolster forward and underneath your knees. Reach one arm overhead, then roll to that side and rest with your head cradled on your upper arm. Slowly sit up.

2. Place the props for **Supported Supine Spinal Twist (p. 130)** and enter the twist with your left hip and left shoulder on the floor. Breathe naturally for 2 minutes 30 seconds, then close the arms until you arrive back fully on your left side. Keep a gentle squeeze of the blanket between your knees as you roll onto your back. Move the bolster to the other side of the mat, then drop your knees and arms to the right and repeat the pose on this side for 2 minutes 30 seconds.

....

TRANSITION: Remove the blanket from your knees and use your hands to sit up.

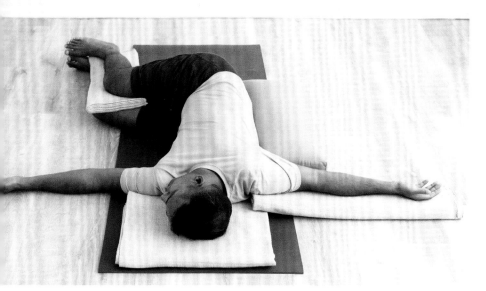

3. Arrange the props for **Supported Child's Pose *with ramped bolster* (p. 52)** and come into the pose. Make any minor adjustments until your whole upper body feels totally at ease, then relax the breath completely, staying present to waves of relaxation spreading throughout the scalp, neck, shoulders, and upper back.

....

TRANSITION: Turn your forehead to face the bolster, release your hands from the strap and exhale to sit upright. Move the bolster ramp to the side and come into Table. Stretch your legs back, one at a time, tucking the toes under on the mat.

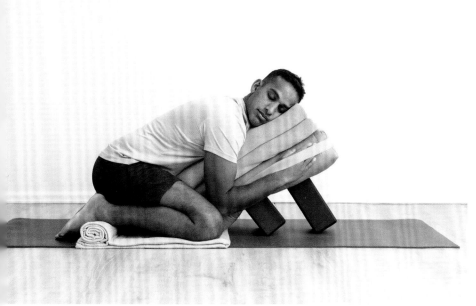

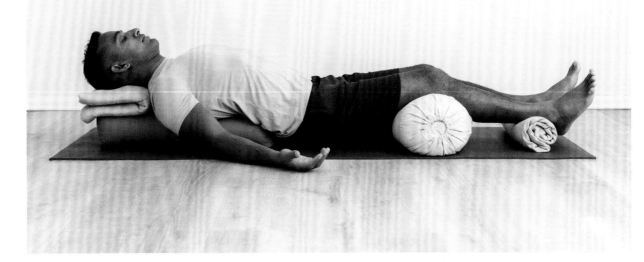

4. Place the props for **Supported Fish (variation) (p. 95)** and enter the pose. Adjust your torso until your spine feels balanced on the bolster and each shoulder may relax outward and downward with gravity. Take care to fully prop your neck for comfort. Practice **Alternate Nostril Breathing Visualization (p. 35)**.

···

TRANSITION: Bend one knee and place the foot on the round bolster. Push the foot down lightly to anchor, then bring the other foot up to the bolster. Roll the bolster away from you, then place your feet flat on the floor. Either carefully roll off to one side or use your hands to slowly sit up.

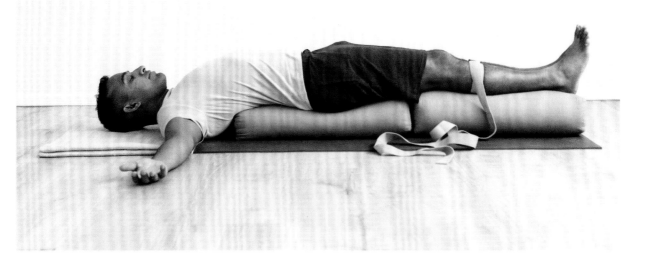

5. Place the props for **Supported Bridge** *with two bolsters* **(p. 104)**. Arrive in the pose and become still, mentally relaxing the pit of the throat and the whole jaw, and softening any creases in your forehead and between your eyebrows. Feel the body decompressing and gaining spaciousness across the chest, shoulders, and arms. *(If you don't have two flat bolsters, you can use one round bolster and one flat bolster.)*

....

TRANSITION: Bend the knees and wiggle backward to slide off the bolster until your hips meet ground. Remove the strap from your legs. Roll to one side and rest for a moment, then slowly sit up.

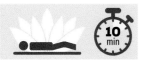

6. Place the props for **Basic Relaxation Pose (p. 37)** and come into the pose. When the body becomes still, just rest and let the breath become effortless.

Promoting a Healthy Spine

TOTAL TIME // 40 MINUTES

WHAT YOU NEED
- Timer
- Mat
- Wall
- Blankets (3–4)
- Blocks (2)
- Flat bolster
- Round bolster
- Looped strap

No matter your age, a good range of spinal movement is essential for maintaining healthy physical well-being. Rejuvenate your spine through side, back, and forward bending, as well as twisting motions, and invite a positive quality, such as "openness," into your body as you practice.

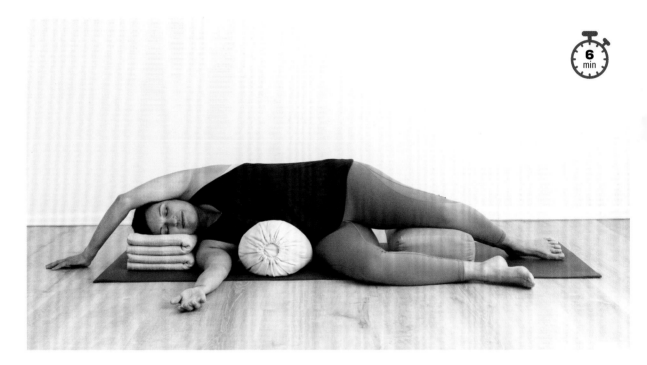

6 min

1. Place the props for **Supported Side-Lying Stretch (p. 126)** and lower your torso down onto your right side to enter the pose. Observe the gentle curve of your spine as it relaxes effortlessly into the props. Rather than forcing a deep breath, allow your breath to ease into a slower, smoother pace. Hold the pose for 3 minutes then lift up sideways from the props and move the flat bolster to the end of the mat. Turn away from the round bolster, sitting on the ground with your feet flat on the floor and knees bent. Widen the feet to the mat's outer edges then drop both knees to the right and then to the left a few times like windshield wipers. End with the knees down so you are sitting on the left hip. Place the bolster back between your legs and repeat on the left side for 3 minutes.

TRANSITION: Press your hands into the floor and exhale to sit up sideways.

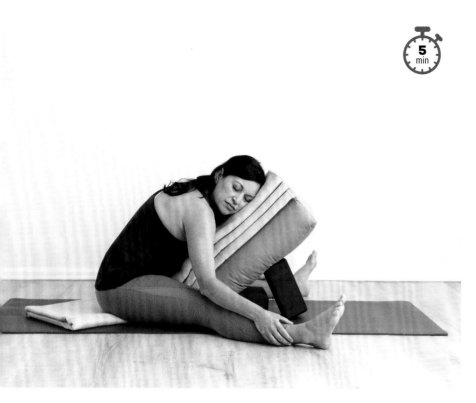

2. Place the props for **Supported Seated Angle (p. 62)** and come into the pose. Release your abdomen fully. Practice **Back Breathing (p. 35)** for 10 rounds.

....

TRANSITION: Exhale and lift your whole spine upright. Place the props that are in front of you off to the side. Use your hands to support under your thighs as you sweep your legs in toward your chest. With knees bent and feet flat on the floor, press your palms into the floor behind you to gently lift the heart upward, softening your shoulder blades down the back. Stay for three easy breaths.

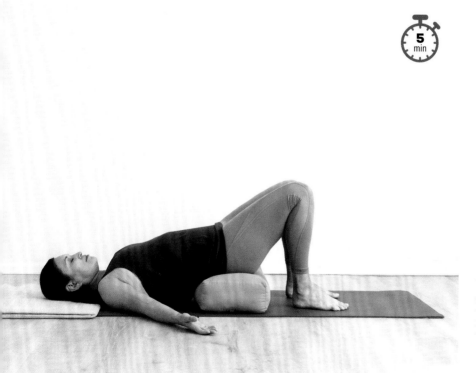

3. Place the props for **Supported Bridge** *with single bolster* **(p. 108)** and lower down into the pose. As you breathe deeper into your abdomen, notice your breath in the low back pressing against the bolster. On your exhales, relax more completely toward the ground and props.

....

TRANSITION: Lift the hips slightly and slide the bolster off the mat so you can rest your hips back to the floor. Cup the knees with the hands and rock gently side to side on the low back. Rest in stillness for three breaths, then roll to one side and sit up.

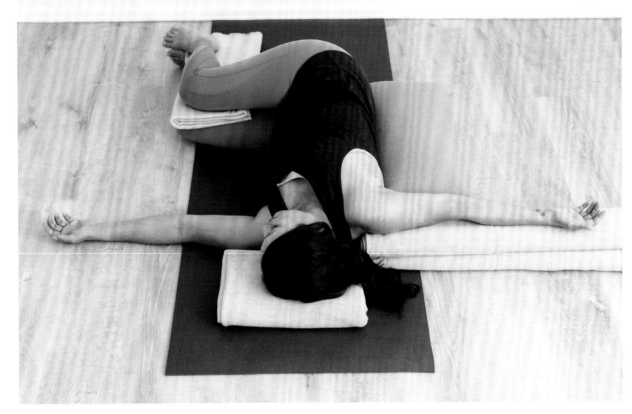

4. Place the props for **Supported Supine Spinal Twist (p. 130)** and lower down into the pose on your left side. Allow the breath to be as it is while staying present to any sensations you may notice. Hold for 2 minutes, then close the arms until you arrive back fully on your side, gazing toward your hands. Keep a gentle squeeze of the blanket between your knees as you roll onto your back. Rest for three breaths. Move the bolster to the other side, then drop your knees and arms to the right and practice the pose on your right side for 2 minutes.

....

TRANSITION: Close the arms together, remove the blanket from your knees, and use your hands to slowly sit up.

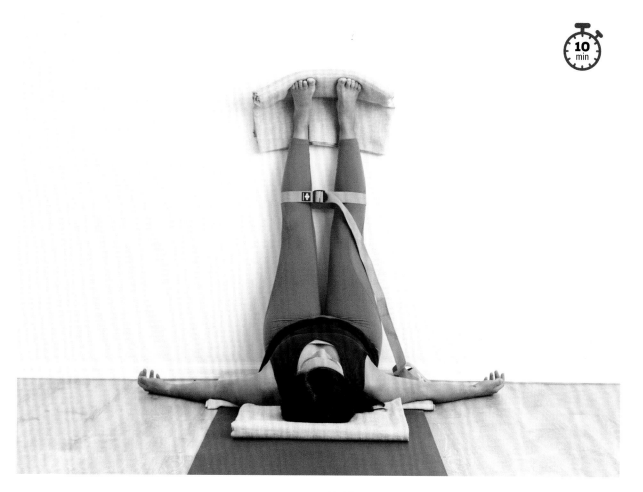

5. Place the props for **Legs Up the Wall (p. 114)** and come into the pose. For extra comfort, loop a strap around your shins and drape a blanket on top of your feet, behind your heels, and secured against the wall. Practice **Lengthen the Exhale (p. 32)** until you feel content to relax and rest without doing.

....

TRANSITION: Gradually bring movement back into the toes and fingers. Slide the feet down the wall, remove the blanket and strap if using, then reach one arm overhead and roll to that side. Rest for a moment before sitting up and moving away from the wall.

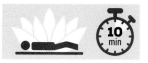

6. Place the props for **Basic Relaxation Pose (p. 37)** and enter the pose. If desired, rest the soles of your feet against the wall to feel grounded and stable in your spine. Recall your positive quality and trust that it is with you now.

Easing Insomnia and Welcoming Deeper Sleep

TOTAL TIME // 40 MINUTES

WHAT YOU NEED
- Timer
- Mat
- Wall
- Blankets (5)
- Blocks (2)
- Flat bolster
- Hand towel
- Looped strap
- Eye pillow (optional)

Add this peaceful practice to your self-care bedtime routine to help restore your body's natural sleep rhythm. Close your eyes and envision a container, then imagine exhaling all your worries about sleep into that container. Seal the container and set it aside to begin your practice.

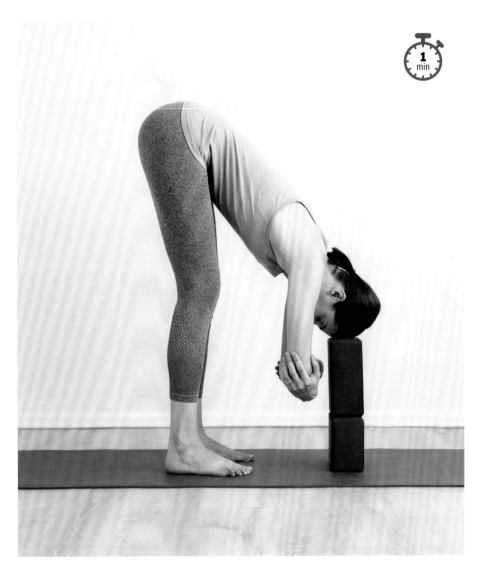

1 min

1. Place the props for **Supported Standing Forward Bend (p. 68)** and enter the pose. Practice **Open Mouth Exhale with Mantra (p. 35),** taking generous breaths in through the nose and out through the mouth while feeling the upper body growing heavier and heavier.

TRANSITION: Instead of standing all the way up, lift your head up from the blocks and place your hands on top of the blocks to steady yourself as you walk your feet back, bend your knees, and come down into Table on the mat. Remove the blocks from the mat and practice three slow rounds of Cow and Cat Pose, feeling your spine unwind any tension from the day.

2. Place the props for **Supported Reclining Bound Angle (p. 86)** and recline back into the pose. Before entering stillness, place your left hand on your heart and your right hand on your abdomen, and connect with the movement of both these places for three gentle rounds of breath. Sense your body letting go even more, then move your arms by your sides and just breathe naturally (*if Supported Reclining Bound Angle with ramped bolster is more comfortable, choose it instead*).

TRANSITION: Lift your knees together to touch, then extend your legs long in front of you and slowly sit up.

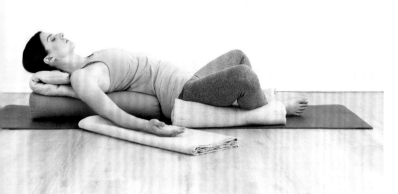

3. Place the props for **Supported Supine Spinal Twist (p. 130)** and lie on your left hip and shoulder to begin the twist. Breathe naturally, observing any gentle opening you may feel across your chest. Hold for 2 minutes, then close your arms together. Gently squeeze the blanket between your knees and roll onto your back, with feet landing on the floor and knees bent. Move the bolster to the other side of the mat. Roll onto your right hip and shoulder to repeat the twist on this side for 2 minutes.

TRANSITION: Close the arms together, remove the blanket from your knees, and use your hands to slowly sit up.

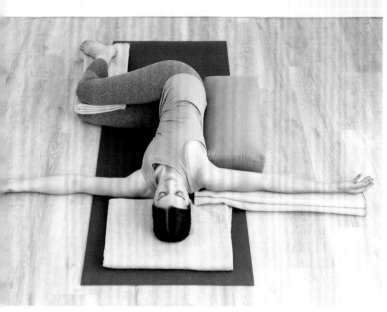

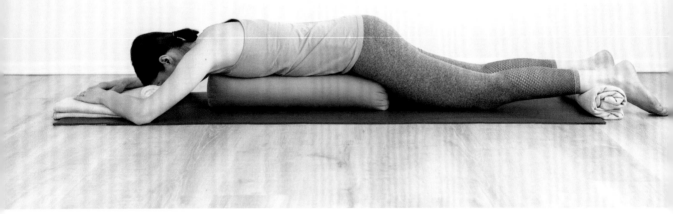

4. Place the props for **Surfboard (p. 54)** and come into the pose. Become aware of the pause in between each breath you take, feeling the abdomen expand and contract against the bolster. Relax your face and jaw completely.

....

TRANSITION: Place your palms on the floor and at the sides of the bolster, then exhale and press up into Table.

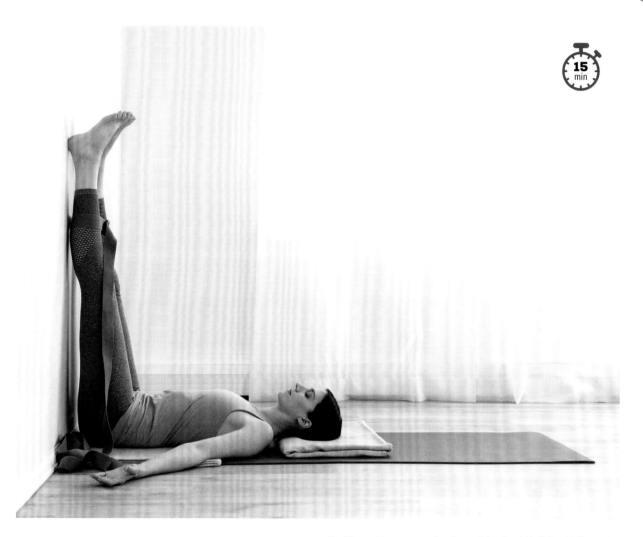

5. Place the props for **Legs Up the Wall (p. 114)** and come into the pose. If necessary, loop the strap loosely around the calves, and apply the eye pillow, if it's comfortable. With steady, even breath, simultaneously soften the skin of your feet and the palms of your hands, and release tension from the tongue and jaw. Sense relaxation in the meeting place of the legs and hips. Let the breath and the body be.

TRANSITION: Exhale, walk your feet down the wall and roll to one side. Rest for a few breaths. Remove the strap if using and take your time to sit up.

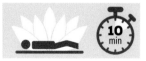

6. Place the props for **Basic Relaxation Pose (p. 37)** and come into the pose. If it's comfortable, apply the eye pillow to further decrease your sense of sight, allowing you to ease into a more restful sleep after your practice is complete. Become aware of the increased sense of quiet in your mind.

Recovery from Exhaustion & Fatigue

TOTAL TIME // 45 MINUTES

WHAT YOU NEED
- Timer
- Mat
- Wall
- Blankets (7)
- Block
- Flat bolster
- Round bolster
- Looped strap (optional)
- Eye pillow (optional)

When the body speaks through fatigue—whether due to a health condition or to diet and lifestyle choices—this sequence is a refuge. Release all expectations to overcome fatigue and just allow yourself to be exactly as you are. Repeat the mantra "I am" to remain present.

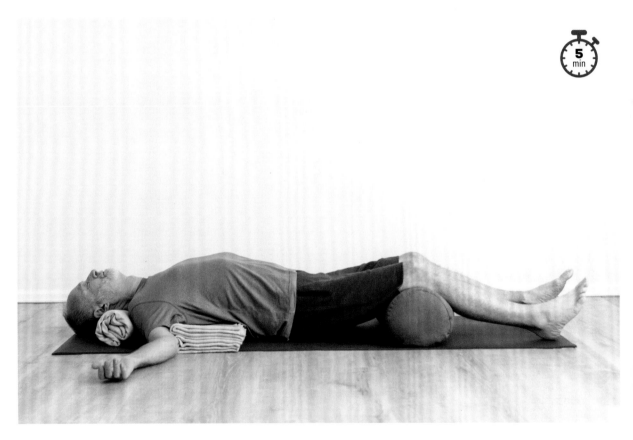

5 min

1. Place the props for **Mountain Brook (p. 84)** and enter the pose. Take three rounds of intentional, deeper breath to ease your way into stillness—inhaling through the nose, while emphasizing a longer exhale through the back of an open mouth—then relax the face and just breathe naturally.

....

TRANSITION: Bend your knees slowly, one at a time, placing your feet on the bolster. Roll the bolster away from you, then curl onto one side for a moment to rest. Sit up slowly.

2. Place the props for **Supported Wheel (variation) (p. 111)** and come into the pose. Bathe yourself in a slow, continuous stream of inhale and exhale so that the breath becomes a never-ending circle. *(It may be helpful to visualize inhaling like a crescent arc on the front of the body, from the tailbone to the base of the neck, then exhaling the other half of the arc down the back body to the tailbone.)*

....

TRANSITION: Release the control of your breath. Press into the feet to slide your upper body backward until only the hips are on the blankets, then roll to one side to rest before sitting up.

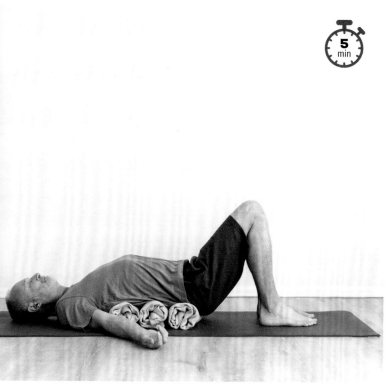

3. Place the props for **Supported Seated Angle (variation) (p. 63)** and come into the pose. Breathe naturally without effort. *(If your knees do not easily touch the floor, pad underneath them with blankets.)*

....

TRANSITION: Bring your hands to hold the bolster, then inhale and lift your head and chest. Set the bolster off to the side. Sweep your legs together, then bend the knees and hug your arms around your legs. Inhale to lengthen your spine upward, then exhale and release the arms.

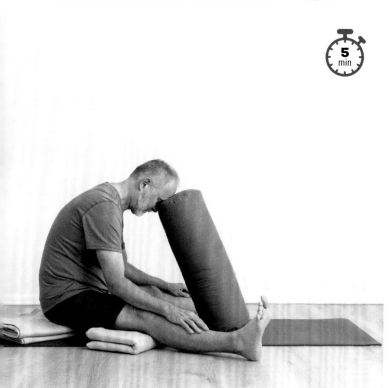

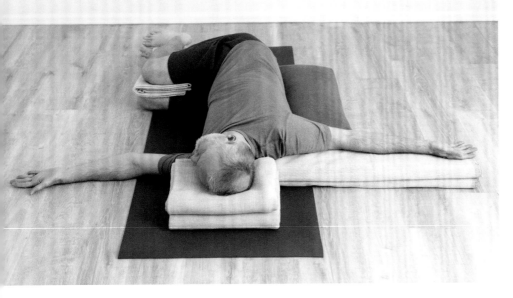

4 min

4. Place the props for **Supported Supine Spinal Twist (p. 130)** then come into the pose on your left hip. Breathe naturally and hold the pose for 2 minutes, then slowly return your arms together and roll onto your back, keeping your knees hugging the blanket and feet flat on the floor. Take a few slow breaths, then move the bolster to the other side of the mat. Lower down to your right hip and repeat the pose on the this side for 2 minutes.

TRANSITION: Close the arms together, remove the blanket from your knees, and use your hands to slowly sit up.

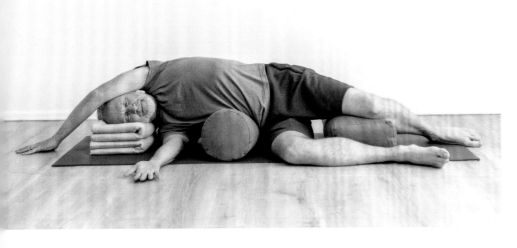

6 min

5. Place the props for **Supported Side-Lying Stretch (p. 126)** and come into the pose on your right hip. Bring your attention to the nostril that is closest to the ceiling, sensing the breath flowing through this nostril and into the lung on that side of the body. Hold the pose for 3 minutes, then slowly press upright, turn away from the round bolster as you lift your knees up and drop them to your left to sit on your left hip. Repeat the pose on this side for 3 minutes.

TRANSITION: Press your hands into the floor and exhale to slowly sit up sideways.

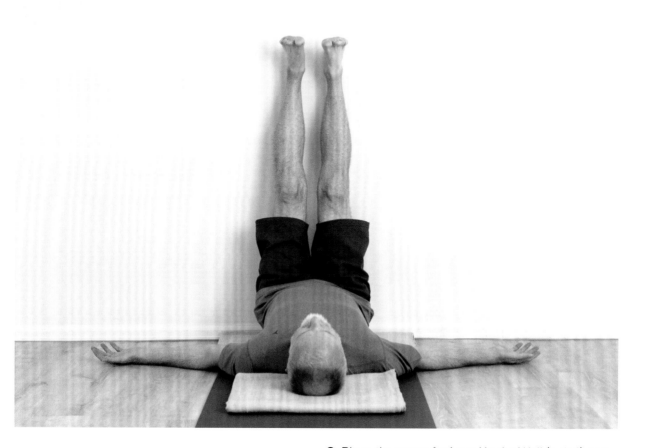

6. Place the props for **Legs Up the Wall (p. 114)** and come into the pose. Once you've arrived, give the breath over to its natural rhythm.

....

TRANSITION: Exhale and walk your feet down the wall. Open the knees outward, leaving the outer edges of the feet against the wall and pressing the soles of the feet together, or crossing your feet at the ankles. Rest for a few breaths in this position, then drop the knees and feet down to one side before slowly sitting up.

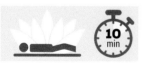

7. Place the props for **Side-Lying Relaxation Pose (p. 39)** and come into the pose on your left side. Practice a moment of gratitude, naming one thing you are grateful for receiving through your practice. For example, "I am grateful for the opportunity to slow down and heal." Release all thought and rest.

Calming Anxiety & Worry

TOTAL TIME // 35 MINUTES

Anxiety and worry are projections of possible problems that could happen in the future. To reclaim the present moment, set an intention to be with what's tangibly happening now in each pose. Use a simple mantra such as, "I am here now," or "Only this is happening now."

WHAT YOU NEED
- Timer
- Mat
- Blankets (4)
- Blocks (2)
- Flat bolster
- Round bolster
- Hand towel
- Eye pillow (optional)

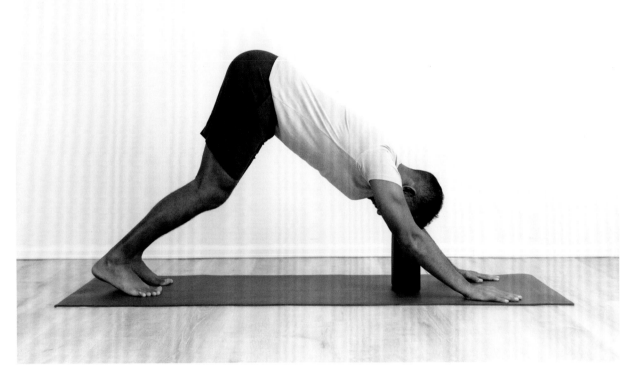

1. Place the props for **Supported Downward-Facing Dog (p. 42)** and enter the pose. Let the breath be quiet and fluid, and feel your muscles engaging just enough to hold the pose.

TRANSITION: Exhale, drop your knees to the ground and rest cross-legged or on your heels, feeling a lightness in your headspace.

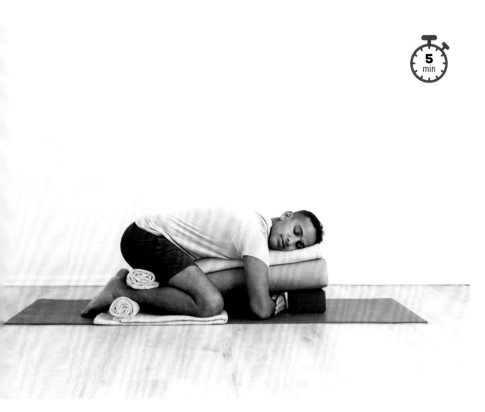

2. Place the props for **Supported Child's Pose (p. 46)** and come into the pose. *(If the regular pose is too uncomfortable, try the variation shown here.)* Practice **Back Breathing (p. 35)** for 10 rounds of breath, counting down from 10 to 1, then relax and just breathe naturally. *(For additional comfort, place a basic-fold blanket across your hips and low back, letting your body yield to the blanket's gentle weight.)*

....

TRANSITION: Push through the palms to slowly rise up into Table. Stretch one leg back at a time.

3. Place the props for **Surfboard (p. 54)** and come into the pose. Feel the comforting connection of your belly against the bolster, and observe your breath moving in and out. *(For additional comfort, fold a blanket just twice and drape it across your back and hips.)*

....

TRANSITION: Return to Table and practice one slow round of Cow and Cat, noticing the quality of your mind and breath.

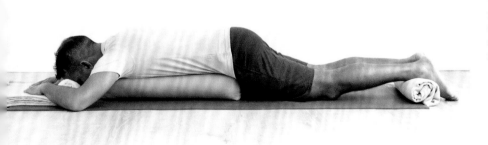

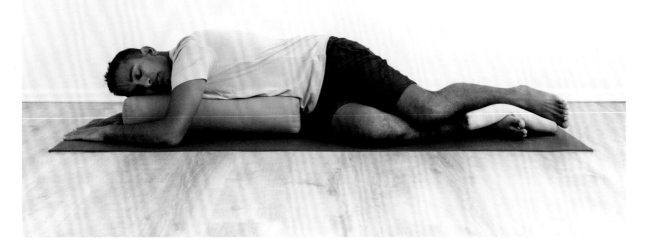

4. Place the props for **Supported Spinal Twist (p. 128)** and come into the pose on your right hip, releasing all effort in the breath. Hold for 3 minutes then, moving slowly, rise to seated as you unwind the twist. Keep your knees hugged together as you turn to the opposite side to repeat the pose for 3 minutes. *(If find your mind wandering into the future, use the intention you created before the practice to bring your mind back.)*

TRANSITION: Slowly sit up, turning to face away from the bolster to stretch out your legs in front of you. Take a moment to pause and enjoy a deep inhale and exhale.

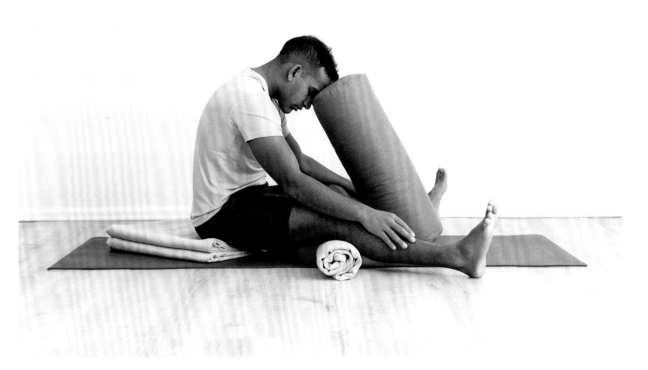

5. Place the props for **Supported Seated Angle (variation) (p. 63)** and come into the pose. Once the body is fully comfortable, the mind will follow. Practice **Lengthen the Exhale (p. 32)** feeling stressors, worries, and troubles releasing from the headspace, traveling down the spine, into the ground, and deep into the earth below. *(For additional comfort, wrap a basic-fold blanket around your low back and around the tops of your thighs.)*

....

TRANSITION: Hold the bolster with your hands, then inhale and lift your head and chest. Set the bolster off to the side and bring your legs together, feeling lighter and more spacious.

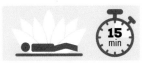

6. Place the props for **Wrapped Relaxation Pose (p. 36)** and come into the pose. Repeat your simple mantra to yourself, feeling that it is enough in this moment to just be here and let go of all physical and mental effort.

Awakening Vitality

TOTAL TIME // 45 MINUTES

As you begin this practice, reflect for a few moments on what it would feel like to embody peaceful, vital energy in your life more often, then create a present-tense, positive statement that embodies this feeling. For example, "I experience good health and a calm, focused mind."

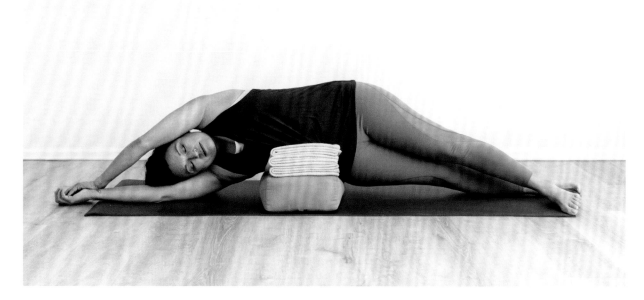

1. Place the props for **Side-Lying Stretch (p. 122)** and enter the pose on your right hip. As you reach through your limbs, expand the breath actively into the ribcage on inhale, and let the body relax into the props on exhale. Hold for 2 minutes, then drop your right hip to the floor as you lift up sideways to seated. Take one full, complete breath, then rotate around to sit on your left hip and complete the pose on this side for 2 minutes.

TRANSITION: Slowly drop your hip to the floor and sit up.

2. Place the props for **Supported Bridge** *with two bolsters* (p. 104) and come into the pose. Practice **Open Mouth Exhale with Mantra** (p. 35) for 10 rounds, then just breathe naturally.

....

TRANSITION: Bend your knees, slide backward off the bolsters, and remove the strap from the legs. Roll to one side and rest for a few breaths, then press up into seated.

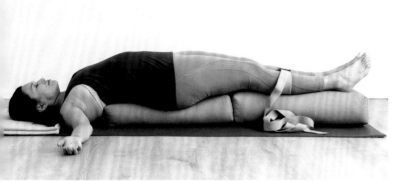

3. Place the props for **Supported Supine Spinal Twist (variation)** (p. 133) and come into the pose, maintaining continuous, easy, and natural breath. Hold the pose for 3 minutes, then close the right arm to come out of the twist. Hug the blanket between your knees and lift them upward, resting with your hips and low back fully on the bolster and feet flat on the ground, then scoot your right hip underneath you and drop your knees to the right to repeat the twist on this side for 3 minutes.

....

TRANSITION: Roll again to your back, then slide backward off the bolster until your hips meet the ground. Rest for a moment before dropping your knees to one side, then sit up slowly.

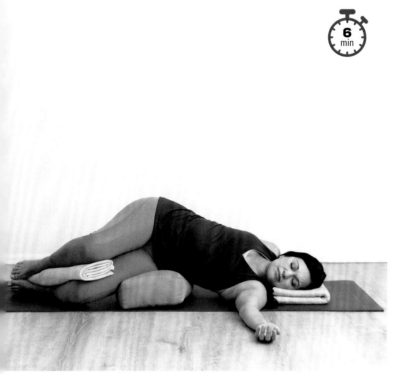

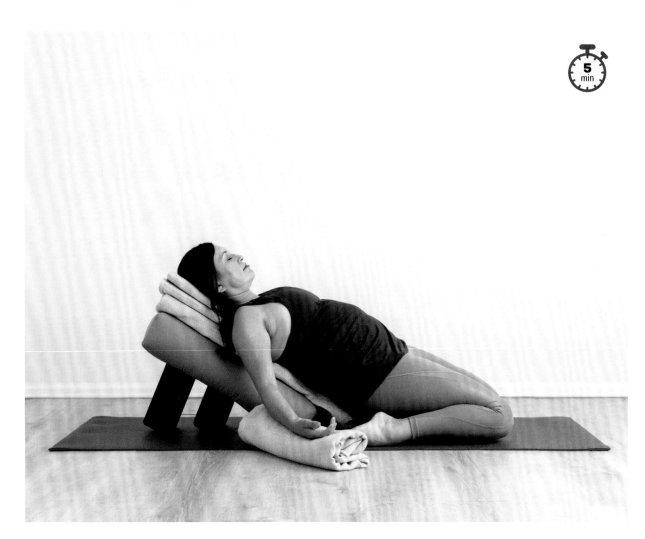

4. Place the props for **Supported Reclining Hero (variation with ramped bolster) (p. 99)** and lower back into the pose. Stay present with the gentle movement of breath in the abdomen and chest areas. If desired, practice **Lengthen the Exhale (p. 32)** to help calm a busy mind.

TRANSITION: Exhale and rise forward into Table, stretching your legs back one at a time.

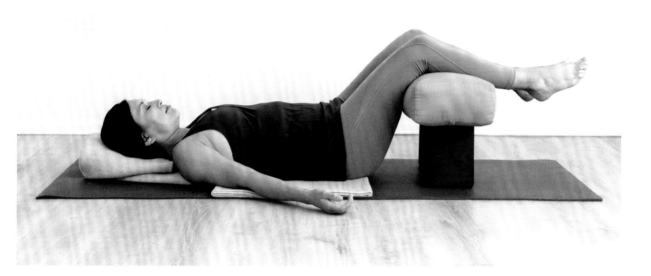

5. Place the props for **Stonehenge (p. 138)** and come into the pose. Do absolutely nothing with the breath, just allow it to settle, becoming still and silent. *(For additional comfort, drape an unfolded blanket over your whole body to stay warm.)*

....

TRANSITION: Moving like molasses, bend your knees one at a time, lifting the legs off the bolster and bringing them toward your heart. Reach one arm overhead and roll to that side. Savor the stillness, using just enough effort to sit up.

6. Place the props for **Basic Relaxation Pose (p. 37)** and enter the pose. Recall your positive statement of vitality, then take three breaths, visualizing on the inhale that this vitality is moving through every cell of your body. As you exhale, release any sensations of dullness or fatigue, then rest in stillness.

Easing Depression

TOTAL TIME // 35 MINUTES

WHAT YOU NEED
- Timer
- Mat
- Wall
- Blankets (2)
- Blocks (3)
- Flat bolster
- Looped strap (optional)
- Eye pillow (optional)

I first came to yoga because of depression, and I came out of depression because of yoga. To regain connection with your true nature, imagine a beautiful place where you're at ease, soothed, and peaceful. Experience yourself fully in this inner sanctuary for one minute, then begin.

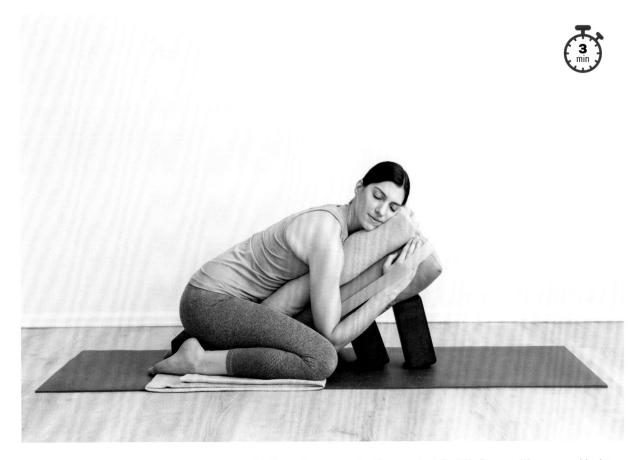

3 min

1. Place the props for **Supported Child's Pose** *with ramped bolster* **(p. 52)** and lower down into the pose. Feel your body being received by the props like a warm hug, with hands nestled under the strap, as you become aware of the breath moving in and out of the nostrils.

TRANSITION: Release your hands to the floor, then use gentle effort to rise into a seat. Move your bolster ramp to the side, then come into Table and stretch your legs back one at a time.

2. Place the props for **Supported Bridge** *with single bolster* **(p. 108)** and come into the pose. Practice **Lengthen the Exhale (p. 32)** until you feel a natural willingness of the breath to settle into a deeper, softer rhythm. Let the breath breathe you.

....

TRANSITION: Maintain relaxation in your face as you lift your hips and slide the bolster to the side, then return with your whole spine on the floor. Bring the knees toward the heart and then roll to one side, resting for a breath before sitting up.

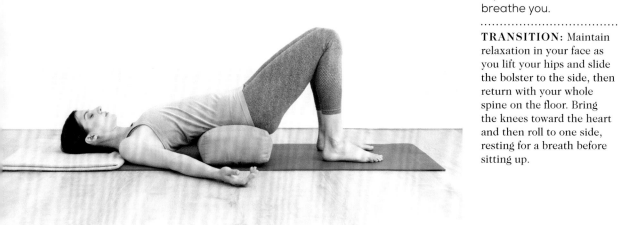

3. Place the props for **Supported Standing Wide-Legged Forward Bend (p. 58)** and come into the pose on a long exhale. Breathe smoothly, feeling the warmth that may pool in your face.

....

TRANSITION: With hands on your hips, raise the whole spine at once to standing. Step your legs inward and become aware of any fresh sensations arriving in the head and heart.

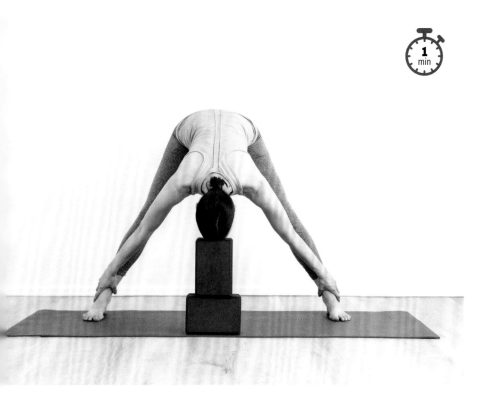

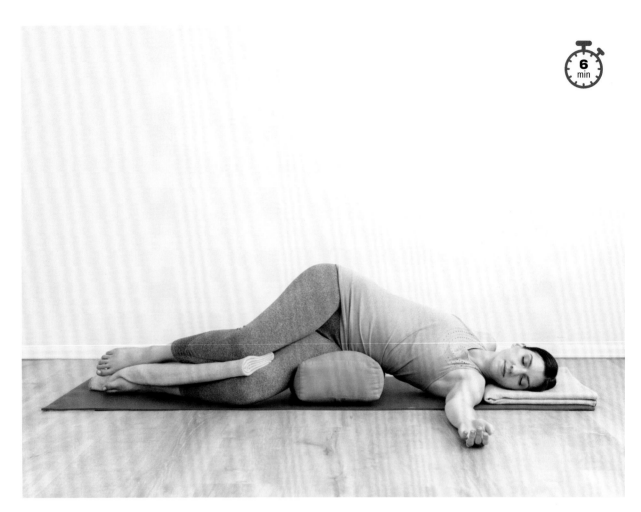

4. Place the props for **Supported Supine Spinal Twist (variation) (p. 133)**. Breathe naturally, perhaps returning to your inner sanctuary. Hold for 3 minutes, then keep the blanket hugged between your knees as you roll onto your back with your hips resting on the bolster and feet on the mat. Turn to the right hip and drop your knees down to repeat the twist on this side for 3 minutes.

TRANSITION: Roll onto your back once more, then slide backward off the bolster until your hips meet the ground. Rest for a moment before dropping your knees to one side, then slowly sit up.

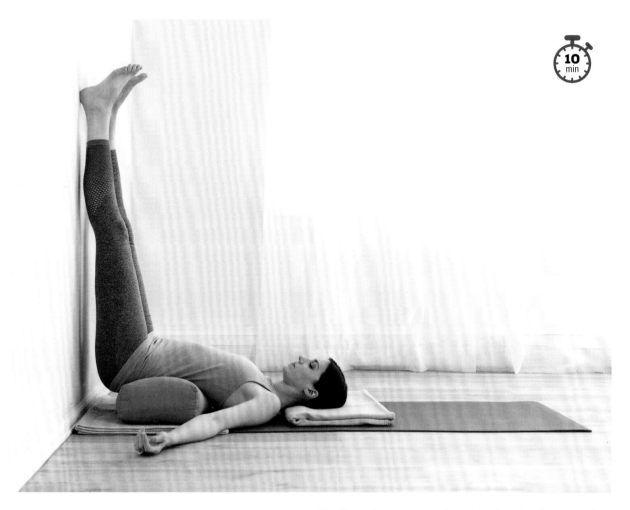

5. Place the props for **Legs Up the Wall (variation) (p. 117)** and come into the pose. If using, add the looped strap around the calves. Breathe easily into the fullness of your lungs, welcoming spaciousness and lightness in your legs and entire body.

....

TRANSITION: Exhale and slowly walk your feet down the wall, bending your knees toward your heart, then carefully roll off the bolster and to one side. Take a moment for your legs to adjust, then sit up.

6. Place the props for **Basic Relaxation Pose (p. 37)** and enter the pose. Recall your inner sanctuary, then drop the visual and absorb yourself in the feeling of being okay exactly as you are. Release all effort as you rest.

Soothing Stress

TOTAL TIME // 40 MINUTES

When stressed, we tend to speed up our thoughts, words, and actions, leading us to do or say things we normally wouldn't. Name your source of stress specifically in the third person. For example, "<your name> is experiencing stress about...." Carry that awareness into the practice.

WHAT YOU NEED
- Timer
- Mat
- Wall
- Blankets (4–5)
- Blocks (2)
- Flat bolster
- Round bolster
- Eye pillow (optional)

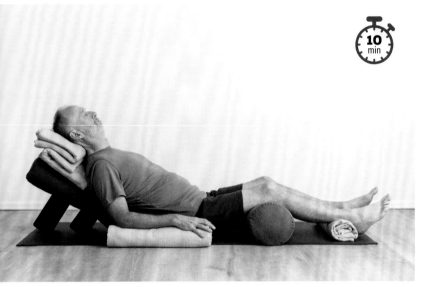

10 min

1. Place the props for **Supported Reclining Pose (p. 90)** and enter the pose. To feel more grounded, leave the blankets and arms on the floor rather than propped on your thighs. Bring your awareness to your chest and abdominal regions. Without strain, practice **Equal Breathing (p. 32)**.

TRANSITION: Dissolve the breathing practice and return to effortlessness in the whole torso. Use your hands to slowly sit up.

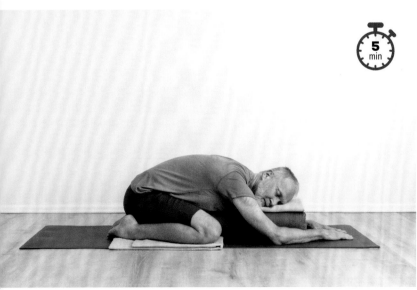

5 min

2. Place the props for **Supported Child's Pose (p. 46)** and lower down into the pose. Relax all effort in the breath, feeling burdens and worries wash off your shoulders.

TRANSITION: Press lightly into your palms to raise the head above the heart. Pause for a few easy breaths in Table, stretching the legs back one at a time.

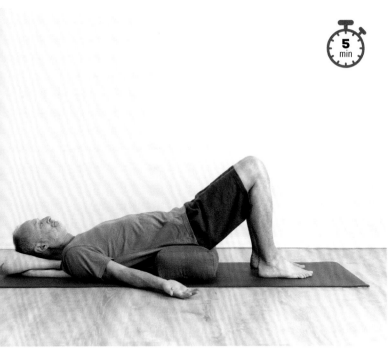

3. Place the props for **Supported Bridge** *with single bolster* **(p. 108)** and recline back into the pose. Expand the ribs with a deeper breath in, then slowly exhale through the nose, allowing the shoulder blades to become spacious on the floor. Breathe naturally.

....

TRANSITION: Remove the bolster, then savor the feeling of hugging your legs in toward your heart with your whole back on the floor. Roll to one side, pausing for a breath, before sitting up.

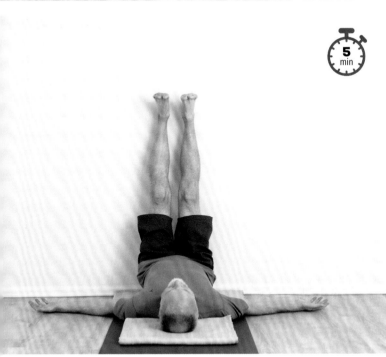

4. Place the props for **Legs Up the Wall (p. 114)** and come into the pose. Become aware of the spaciousness in your abdomen and softness in your skin. Breathe naturally, visualizing the breath moving beyond the boundaries of the lungs and into the whole body.

....

TRANSITION: Exhale, then walk your feet down the wall and roll to one side. Rest here, then slowly sit up.

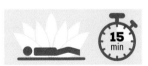

5. Place the props for **Basic Relaxation Pose (p. 37)** and come into the pose. Once still, ask yourself, "What am I experiencing now?" Notice if the answer is different than what you were feeling at the start of the practice, then let go and receive the nourishing silence.

Deeper Breathing

TOTAL TIME // 40 MINUTES

WHAT YOU NEED
- Timer
- Mat
- Blankets (5–6)
- Flat bolster
- Round bolster
- Looped strap
- Eye pillow (optional)

Breathing has a powerful effect on the state of your body, mind, and energy. Better breathing starts by becoming aware of how you're currently inhaling and exhaling. Is it full or shallow? Smooth or rough? Tuck this self-discovery away for later and begin the sequence.

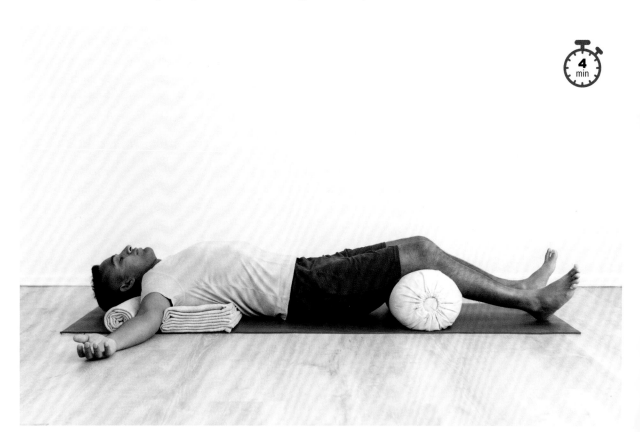

4 min

1. Place the props for **Mountain Brook (p. 84)** and come into the pose, sensing your body rippling like a gentle wave over the support. Release all doing and enter being, attuning yourself to the natural rhythm of your breath as if you are floating on a raft; feel the inhales lift your body, and exhale as the wave passes you by. Take your time and breathe without effort or strain, just float in the still space between the waves.

TRANSITION: Release the visualization of the breath, then slowly begin to move your fingers and toes. Bend your knees, roll the bolster away from your legs, and curl up on your side. Rest for a moment before sitting up.

2. Place the props for **Side-Lying Stretch (p. 122)** and come into the pose on your right hip. Feel as if you are breathing fully into the left lung and left rib cage as you hold the position.

TRANSITION: Drop your right hip to the floor as you lift up sideways to seated. Breathe in clearly through the nose, filling up both lungs, then exhale and release all air. Staying on your hip, rearrange the props so that you can simply lie down on the floor and continue with the next pose.

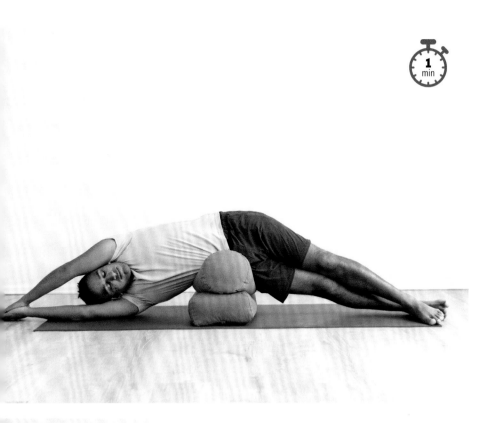

3. Place the props for **Supported Supine Spinal Twist (p. 130)** and come into the pose on your right hip and shoulder, opening your left arm into the twist. Relax your jaw, tongue, and lips, sensing openness arising in the left side of the chest. Do absolutely nothing to the breath other than observing where it lives in your body.

TRANSITION: Close your arm to come out of the twist. Press your palms into the floor and rise into a seat, with legs crossed or extended. Pause to observe any shifts in the left side of the body compared to the right side of the body.

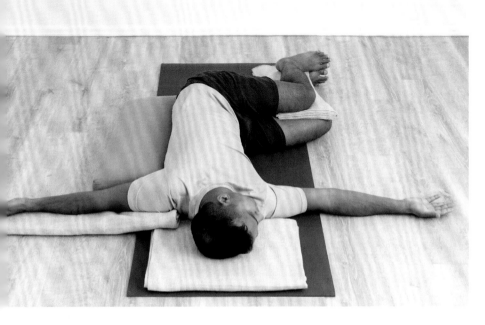

4. Place the props once again for **Side-Lying Stretch (p. 122)**, but this time enter the pose on your left hip. Feel as if you are breathing fully into the right lung and right rib cage.

TRANSITION: Drop your left hip to the floor as you lift your torso up. Take a clearing breath through the nose, expanding the chest, then exhale and empty fully, staying on your left hip so you can rearrange the props and continue with the next pose.

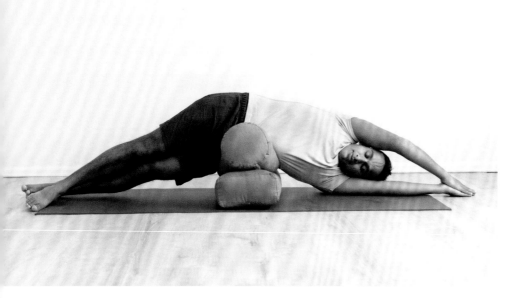

5. Reposition once again for **Supported Supine Spinal Twist (p. 130)** and come into the pose on your left hip and shoulder, opening your right arm into the twist. Observe the breath without controlling it.

TRANSITION: Close your arm to come out of the twist. Press your palms into the floor and rise to a seat, perhaps with your legs crossed or extended. Pause to observe any shifts in the right side of the body compared to the left side of the body.

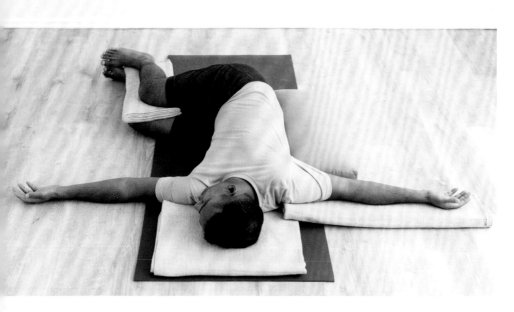

6. Place the props for **Supported Reclining Bound Angle (p. 86)** and come into the pose. Before settling into stillness, place your right hand on your abdomen and your left hand on your heart, and take three deep breaths. Feel your hands rise and fall gently, then release your hands into the pose and just breathe naturally.

TRANSITION: Lift your knees together to touch, then extend your legs long in front of you. Press the palms into the floor to slowly sit up.

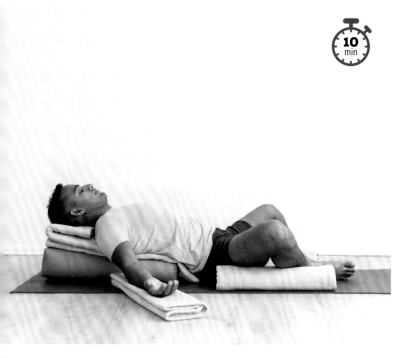

7. Place the props for **Supported Bridge *with two bolsters* (p. 104)** and come into the pose, looping the strap around your calves before lying back onto the bolster. Do nothing to the breath but observe it moving in and out, perhaps noticing if there is a coolness or warmth on your upper lip.

TRANSITION: Bend your knees, slide backward off the bolsters, and loosen the strap from your legs. Roll to one side and rest for a few breaths, then slowly sit up.

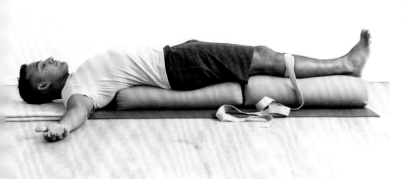

8. Place the props for **Basic Relaxation Pose *with chest elevated* (p. 38)** and come into the pose. Notice if the way your breath is moving in your body feels more spacious compared to when you began, then release all effort and relax.

Grounding During Change

TOTAL TIME // 40 MINUTES

Change is an opportunity for self-reflection—to see from where you've come and to where you might go. This sequence is a soft landing for you to navigate emotions and thoughts around transitions. Let the earth hold you as you lay down your responsibilities and become present.

WHAT YOU NEED
- Timer
- Mat
- Wall
- Blankets (3)
- Block
- Flat bolster
- Hand towel
- Looped strap
- Eye pillow (optional)

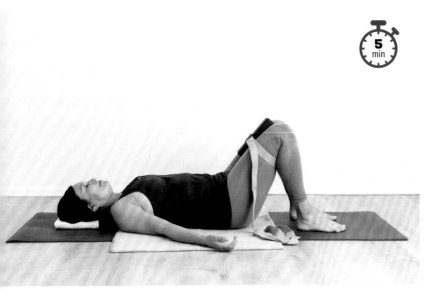

5 min

1. Place the props for **Constructive Rest Position (p. 80)** and come into the pose. Tell your body it's okay to relax its grip in the groins and hips. Practice **Equal Breathing (p. 32)**, filling your lungs to an easy capacity and relaxing even more with the exhalations.

TRANSITION: Remove the props from your legs, then slowly slide your heels along the floor while extending the backs of the legs to the ground. Rest for a moment, then bend the knees, roll to a side and sit up.

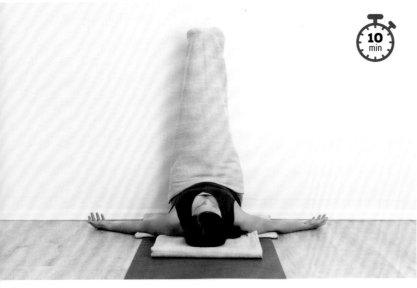

10 min

2. Place the props for **Legs Up the Wall (p. 114)**. Bend your knees, then wrap your legs with a blanket like a cocoon, tucking the ends firmly behind your legs as you straighten your legs back up the wall. Enter stillness. Breathe naturally, opening the arms wide enough to the sides to feel relaxation across the chest.

TRANSITION: Bend your knees and walk your feet down the wall. Remove the blanket, then open the knees wide to each side and either touch the soles of the feet together or cross at the ankles, resting the ankles against the wall. Take three deep breaths. Unwind the legs, close the knees together, and roll to one side. Rest for a moment, then slowly sit up.

3. Place the props for **Supported Bridge** *with single bolster* **(p. 108)** and come into the pose. Take three rounds of deep breath in through the nose, then open the mouth and audibly sigh. Softly close the lips, relax the tongue, and breathe naturally. *(If you feel like yawning, do not suppress it.)*

TRANSITION: Feel the soles of your feet rooted to the earth, then engage your legs, push down into your feet, and lift your hips slightly, using your hands to slide the bolster away so you can rest your hips on the mat. Hug the knees toward your heart, then roll to one side and rest before sitting up.

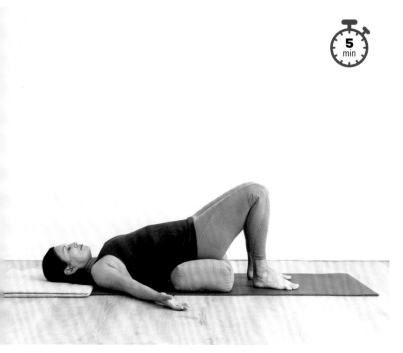

4. Place the props for **Supported Child's Pose (p. 46)** and come into the pose, placing an optional blanket over your hips and lower back area for additional grounding, if desired. Sense the body's heaviness on the floor and the lightness in your natural breath sweeping in and out of the nose. Just be here now.

TRANSITION: Press into your palms to slowly lift your torso upright. Come into Table, stretching one leg back at a time.

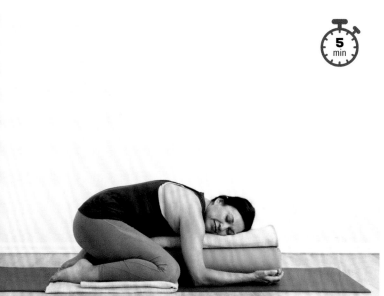

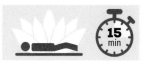

5. Place the props for **Wrapped Relaxation Pose (p. 36)** and come into the pose. To ground yourself in the present moment, silently repeat the mantra "I am here" over the course of three breaths, thinking "I am" on the inhale, and "here" on the exhale, then relax all mental and physical effort and rest.

Relaxation During Pregnancy

TOTAL TIME // 40 MINUTES

Connect deeply with baby and yourself while relieving tension, reducing nausea, and preparing for childbirth. Ask yourself what word you'd like to embody at this time (for example, "gratitude" or "love"). Close your eyes and embrace this quality in your heart, then begin your practice.

WHAT YOU NEED
- Timer
- Mat
- Wall
- Blankets (7)
- Blocks (3)
- Flat bolsters (2)
- Round bolster
- Looped strap (optional)
- Eye pillow (optional)

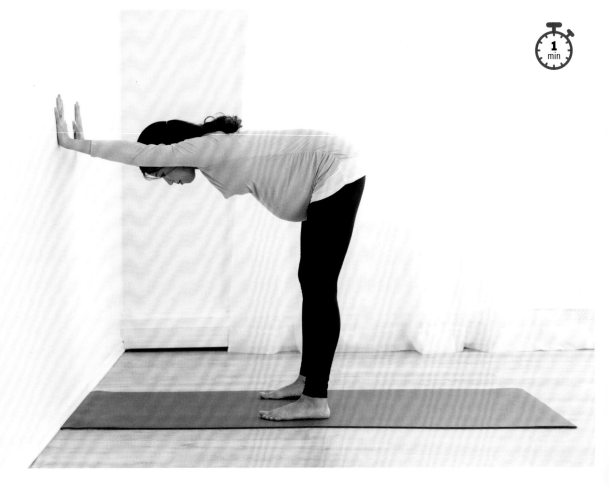

1 min

1. Place the mat for **Half-Dog at Wall (p. 44)** and enter the pose, being careful not to overstretch or hyperextend into your joints. Feel your abdomen descend as you take smooth, long breaths through the nose.

TRANSITION: Inhale as you slowly walk toward the wall while bending your elbows and rising up to stand.

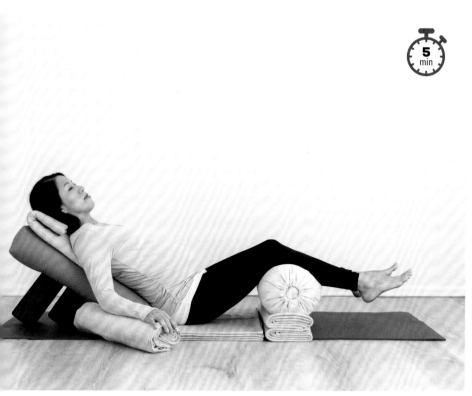

2. Place the props for **Stonehenge** *pregnancy variation* (p. 140). Lower back onto the bolster ramp and check that your heart is elevated higher than your knees. You may choose to place your hands on your abdomen, connecting with your baby and your intention.

TRANSITION: Exhale as you bend your knees, one at a time, and place your feet on top of the round bolster, then roll it away from you. With your feet flat on the mat, use your hands to slowly sit up.

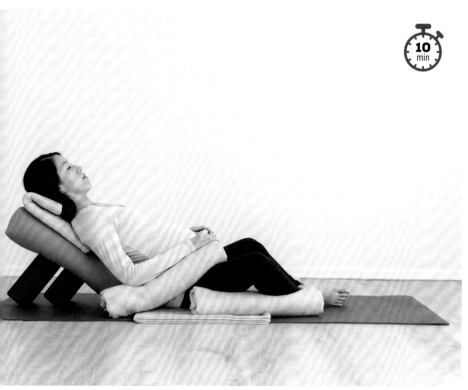

3. Keep the props at your back and remove the bolster and blankets under your legs, then place the remaining props for **Supported Reclining Bound Angle** *with ramped bolster* **(p. 88)**. Lower back onto the props, then settle into the deep comfort of this position, allowing your attention to be drawn toward softer, continuous breath.

TRANSITION: Straighten each leg to the floor, then use your hands to support your upper body into a seat.

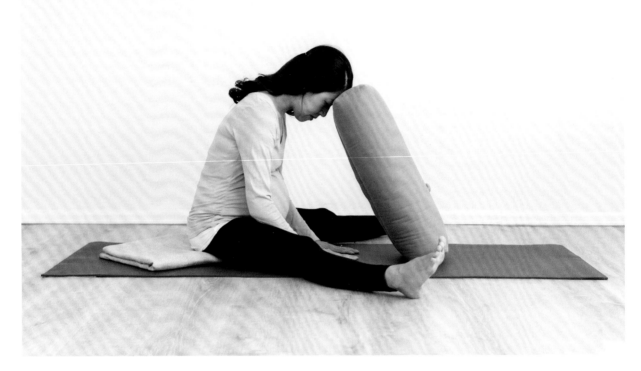

4. Place the props for **Supported Seated Angle (variation) (p. 63)** and enter the pose, allowing your abdomen to slowly drop as you lean forward. Practice **Back Breathing (p. 35)** with ease for 10 rounds.

TRANSITION: Hold the bolster with your hands, then inhale and lift your head and chest. Set the bolster to the side, then collect your legs inward and toward one another, leaving space for your belly.

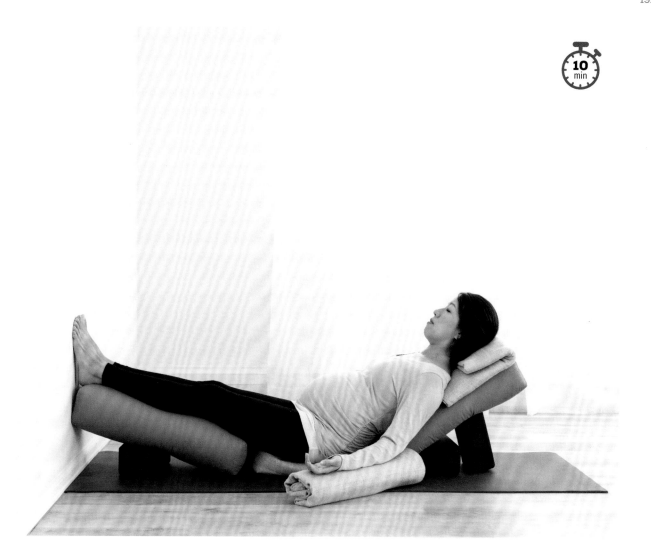

5. Slowly and mindfully place the props for **Legs Up the Wall** *pregnancy variation* **(p. 118)**. Come into the pose, adjusting your feet until they are lightly held against the wall. Relax all effort in the breath and simply be with you and baby.

....

TRANSITION: Begin wiggling the toes and fingers, then bend your knees, place your feet flat on the floor, and slowly inhale as you use your hands to sit up.

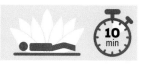

6. Place the props for **Side-Lying Relaxation Pose (p. 39)** and come into the pose, hugging the bolster in front of you. Bring to mind your intention one last time, repeating it silently three times to yourself. Become still and rest.

Promoting Menstrual Health

TOTAL TIME // 30 MINUTES

Practice one week prior to your flow, or when you first notice symptoms of PMS, as prevention for menstrual cramps, plus during your cycle to alleviate fatigue and physical discomfort. During this time of physical shedding, what else might you want to let go of mentally or emotionally?

WHAT YOU NEED
- Timer
- Mat
- Blankets (5)
- Blocks (3)
- Flat bolster
- Looped strap
- Eye pillow (optional)

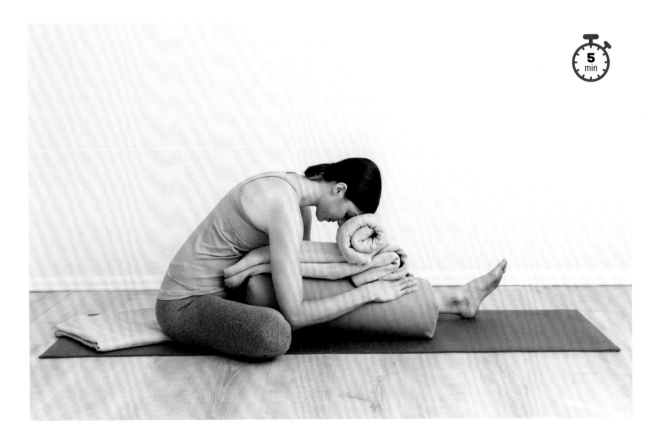

5 min

1. Place the props for **Supported Seated Forward Bend (variation) (p. 75)**. Come into the pose with both legs extended, then bend the right knee while keeping the left leg extended. Practice **Back Breathing (p. 35)**, feeling tension from the head, neck, and shoulders releasing down the spine. Hold for 2 minutes 30 seconds, then lift your torso, reverse the leg positions, and hold for an additional 2 minutes 30 seconds.

TRANSITION: Remove the props from the legs and extend both legs out in front of you.

2. Place the props for **Supported Child's Pose** *with ramped bolster* **(p. 52)**. Lower down into the pose, wrapping an optional blanket around your low back and hips and tucking it into the creases of your thighs for added warmth. Insert your hands into the strap around the bolster and breathe naturally.

TRANSITION: Release your hands from the strap and press into your palms to lift your heart above your hips. Scoot back from the bolster ramp, and from Table, stretch one leg back at a time.

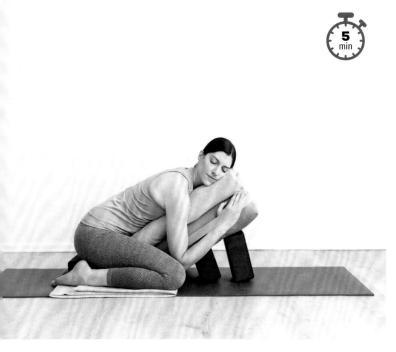

3. Place the props for **Supported Reclining Bound Angle** *with ramped bolster* **(p. 88)**. Exhale and lower your upper body backward and onto the props. Place your palms flat on your abdomen just below your navel, forming a triangle with the tips of your thumbs and index fingers. This is *Trimurti Mudra*, a hand gesture to support reproductive health. Breathe into the space of your abdomen for 10 breaths, then release your arms onto the blankets.

TRANSITION: One at a time, lift a knee up and then extend the leg long in front of you. Remain in this reclined position for a few breaths, then use your hands to slowly sit up.

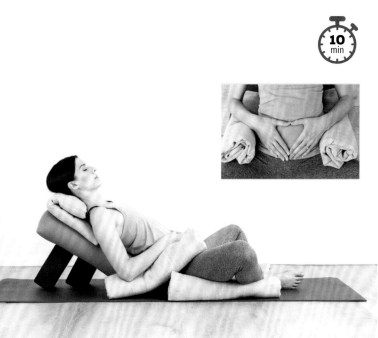

4. Place the props for **Basic Relaxation Pose** *with calves elevated* **(p. 38)** and come into the pose. As you settle deeply into relaxation, use three deep exhalations out of the mouth to release tension and cares from your body and mind, then rest and let the breath become natural.

Easing Symptoms of Perimenopause & Menopause

TOTAL TIME // 45 MINUTES

Embody the true "pause" during this life transition—the still space of peace beneath shifting hormones and symptoms such as fatigue, sleep disturbances, and hot flashes. Call in one helpful attribute, perhaps "patience," to fill your practice with more ease.

WHAT YOU NEED
- Timer
- Mat
- Wall
- Blankets (6)
- Blocks (2)
- Flat bolster
- Looped strap (optional)
- Eye pillow (optional)

NOTE
Do not practice this sequence if you are menstruating.

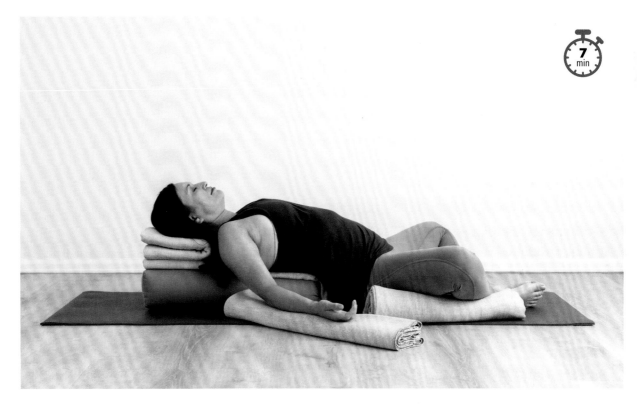

7 min

1. Place the props for **Supported Reclining Bound Angle (p. 86)** and recline into the pose. Practice **Equal Breathing (p. 32)** for as long as you can stay present with it, allowing the breath to become more and more effortless and smooth.

TRANSITION: First extend each leg long onto the floor, then guide your chin toward your chest and exhale as you use your hands to slowly sit up.

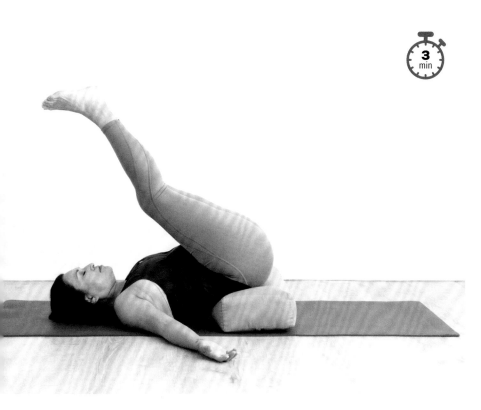

2. Place the props for **Upward-Facing Forward Bend (p. 134)** and come into the pose. Take care to support your sacrum on the bolster, feeling your shoulders heavy on the floor and bending your knees as necessary. Just breathe naturally.

TRANSITION: Slowly lower your feet down to the mat. Wiggle backward from the bolster, resting with it underneath your knees for a few breaths. Curl onto one side, then gradually sit up.

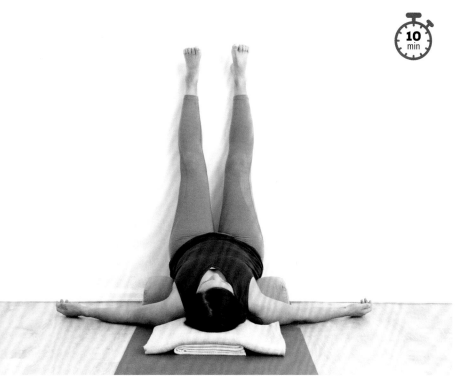

3. Place the props for **Legs Up the Wall (variation) (p. 117)** and come into the pose. If using, loop the strap around your calves. Relax all effort in the breath. There is nothing to do. Just be.

TRANSITION: Exhale as you walk your feet down the wall. With knees bent and feet against the wall, lift the hips and pull the bolster off the mat, then lower your hips to the mat. Pause for a few breaths, then roll to one side and slowly sit up.

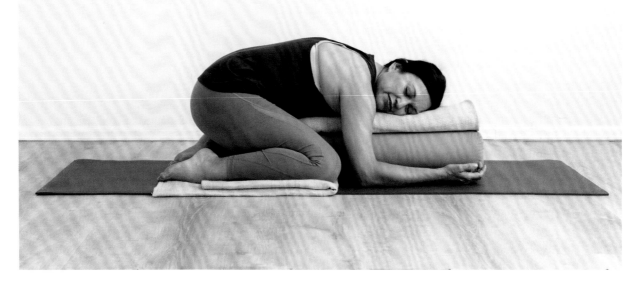

4. Place the props for **Supported Child's Pose (p. 46)**. Lower your abdomen down and feel the energy of movement transform into stillness as you enter the pose. Allow the breath to be easy and natural.

TRANSITION: Use your palms to very slowly press up into seated. Extend your legs back, one at a time, to invigorate the knees and ankles with fresh blood flow.

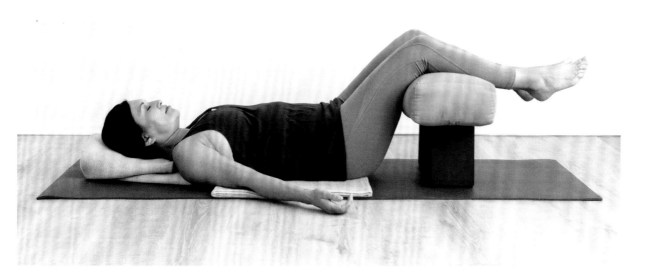

5. Place the props for **Stonehenge (p. 138)** and come into the pose. Practice 10 rounds of **Lengthen the Exhale (p. 32)** then relax the breath completely and rest.

....

TRANSITION: Bend your knees one at a time, lifting the legs off the bolster and bringing them toward your heart. Reach one arm overhead and roll to that side. Pause, then slowly sit up.

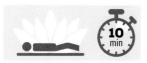

6. Place the props for **Basic Relaxation Pose (p. 37)** and enter the pose. Remember the attribute you invited in at the beginning of practice. Invite that quality to inhabit your whole being as you rest.

Recovery from Traveling & Jet Lag

WHAT YOU NEED
- Timer
- Mat (or bath towel)
- Wall
- Blankets (2)
- Flat bolster (or large pillow)
- Round bolster (or large pillow)

TOTAL TIME // 30 MINUTES

This sequence will help replenish your body and mind, and if needed, you can use items you might find in a hotel room as props. Reflect on one word you would like to plant like a seed into your practice, then frame it as a positive, present tense statement such as, "I am protected."

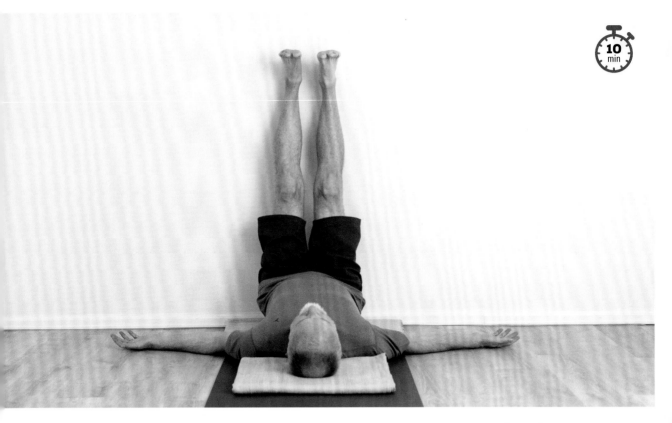

10 min

1. Place the props for **Legs Up the Wall (p. 114)** and enter the pose. Practice **Lengthen the Exhale (p. 32)** for 10 rounds of breath, then let go of all effort in your abdomen, lungs, and throat, and just breathe naturally.

....

TRANSITION: Exhale and walk your feet down the wall. Bend your knees, pull your feet away from the wall, and circle your ankles slowly to encourage blood flow. Roll to one side, rest for a few breaths, then sit up.

2. Place the props for **Supported Bridge** *with single bolster* (p. 108) and come into the pose. Fully support the head so that the neck and shoulders may relax. Observe the gentle movement of the ribs and belly as you breathe naturally.

TRANSITION: Push the feet into the floor to lift the hips slightly, slide the bolster away, then lower your hips to the floor. Roll to one side to rest, then slowly sit up.

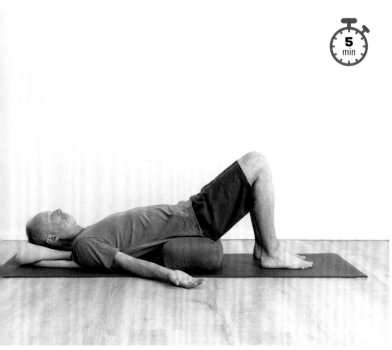

3. Place the props for **Supported Pigeon (p. 64)** and come into the pose. Visualize the breath moving into any areas of tightness or discomfort in your hips from prolonged sitting. Feel spaciousness arrive with the inhalations, and keep that spaciousness as you exhale and tell your muscles to let go. Hold for 2 minutes 30 seconds, then rise to Table and stretch your right leg out behind you. Switch leg positions and repeat on this side for 2 minutes 30 seconds.

TRANSITION: Lift back into Table to stretch the left leg out behind you, then practice three rounds of Cow and Cat Pose.

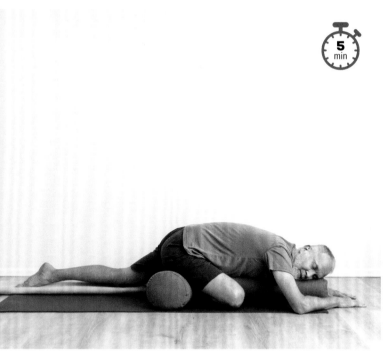

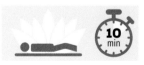

4. Place the props for **Basic Relaxation Pose (p. 37)** and come into the pose. At the gateway of deep rest, repeat your intention three times silently to yourself and feel that it is true in this moment.

Soothing Headaches

TOTAL TIME // 35 MINUTES

It's no secret that stress can contribute to headaches, but did you know that your posture may also be a factor? Find a quiet space, dim the lights, and consider placing an eye pillow or a hand towel around your forehead and ears during this practice.

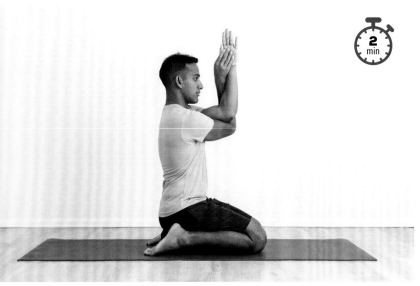

1. Prepare for the restorative poses by standing or sitting on a block and practicing **Eagle Arms Flow (p. 19)**. With slow, full, spacious breath, release any jaw or teeth clenching as you inhale your arms upward and then exhale them down. Practice for 1 minute, then switch the arm positions and repeat on the opposite side for 1 minute.

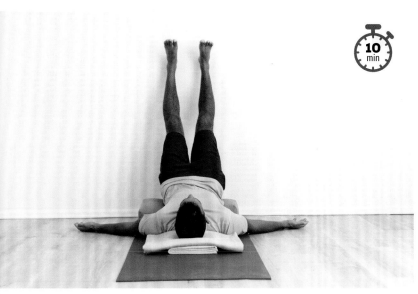

2. Place the props for **Legs Up the Wall (variation) (p. 117)** and come into the pose. Breathe deeply as you bring your hands to the sides of your neck, folding your fingers in toward your palms and using your knuckles to gently massage up and down on the neck muscles. Next use your fingertips to massage up and down and side to side on the jaw joints as you open and close the jaw. Finally, massage the temples and scalp, making circles with gentle pressure. Apply the head covering, if desired.

TRANSITION: Exhale and walk your feet down the wall. With knees bent and feet on the wall, lift the hips and pull the bolster off the mat, then lower your hips down. Pause, then roll to one side and slowly sit up.

3. Place the props for **Supported Reclining Bound Angle** *with ramped bolster* **(p. 88)** and enter the pose. Apply the head covering, if desired. Practice **Longer, Smoother, Softer, Breathing (p. 32)** for 10 rounds, then allow the breath to be natural.

TRANSITION: Become aware of your whole body at peace. One at a time, lift your knees and extend each leg long in front of you, then sit up.

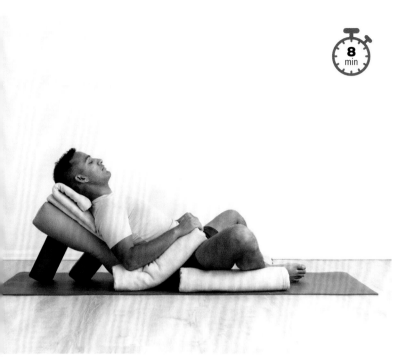

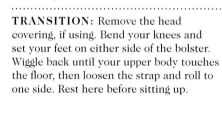

4. Place the props for **Supported Bridge** *with two bolsters* **(p. 104)**. Sit on the bolster, loop the strap over your legs, then lie back into the pose. Apply the head covering, if desired. Observe the natural expansion and contraction of the ribs as you simply allow your body to breathe how it wants. Relax the tongue and the throat.

TRANSITION: Remove the head covering, if using. Bend your knees and set your feet on either side of the bolster. Wiggle back until your upper body touches the floor, then loosen the strap and roll to one side. Rest here before sitting up.

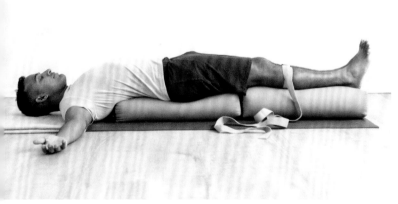

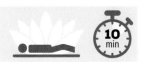

5. Place the props for **Basic Relaxation Pose (p. 37)** and enter the pose. Apply the head or eye covering to block out light and deepen your relaxation. Once you become still, relax any tension in your forehead and the corners of your eyes, then fully let go into the pose.

Index

S